11-10-99

8/11

11/15

MW01107648

DISCARD

MEDICINES
FROM
NATURE

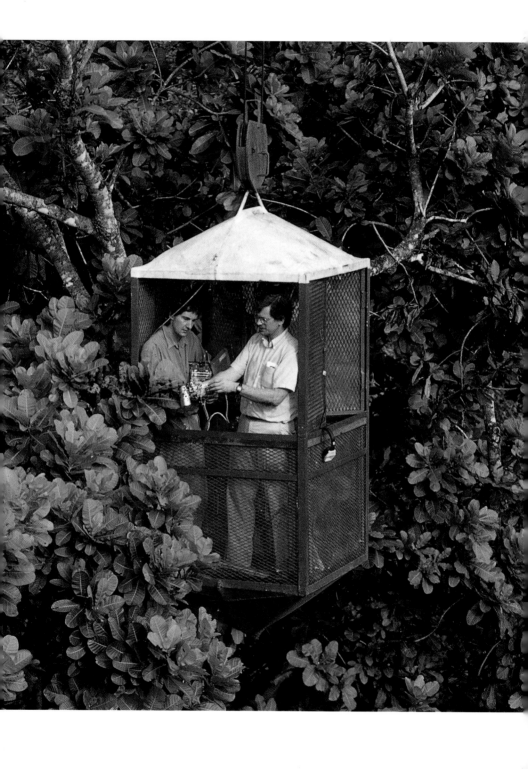

MEDICINES
FROM
NATURE

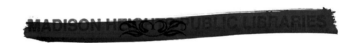

PEGGY THOMAS

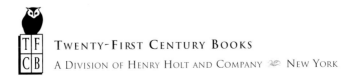

TWENTY-FIRST CENTURY BOOKS
A DIVISION OF HENRY HOLT AND COMPANY ❧ NEW YORK

Twenty-First Century Books
A Division of Henry Holt and Company, Inc.
115 West 18th Street
New York, NY 10011

Henry Holt® and colophon are trademarks of
Henry Holt and Company, Inc.
Publishers since 1866

Published in Canada by Fitzhenry & Whiteside Ltd.
195 Allstate Parkway, Markham, Ontario, L3R 4T8

Library of Congress Cataloging-in-Publication Data
Thomas, Peggy.
Medicines from nature / Peggy Thomas.
p.   cm.
Includes bibliographical references and index.
Summary: Discusses how we have learned from traditional healers
around the world about the medicinal value of substances from nature.
1. Pharmacognosy—Juvenile literature. 2. Ethnobotany—
Juvenile literature. 3. Herbs–Therapeutic use—Juvenile literature.
[1. Drugs. 2. Traditional medicine. 3. Ethnobotany.] I. Title.
RS160.T56 1997
615'.321—dc21   96-47686
                                                                           CIP
                                                                           AC

ISBN 0-8050-4168-0
First Edition—1997

Designed by Kelly Soong

Printed in Mexico
All first editions are printed on acid-free paper ∞.

1 3 5 7 9 10 8 6 4 2

Photo credits
p. 2: ©Gerald Davis/Phototake, Inc.; p. 8: ©Martin Rogers/Woodfin Camp; p. 20:
©Nathan Benn/Woodfin Camp; p. 32: ©H. Morgan/Science Source/Photo Researchers,
Inc.; p. 42: ©Corbis-Bettmann; p.42 (lower left): Andrew McClenaghan/Science Photo
Library/Photo Researchers Inc.; p. 50: ©National Cancer Institute; p. 58: ©Peter K.
Ziminski/Visuals Unlimited; p. 72 (top): ©James Beveridge/Visuals Unlimited; p. 72 (mid-
dle): ©Alese & Mort Pechter/The Stock Market; p. 72 (bottom): ©David M. Barron/
Animals Animals; p. 82 (top): ©George K. Bryce/Animals Animals; p. 82 (middle):
Dr. Jeremy Burgess/Science Photo Library/Photo Researchers Inc.; p. 82 (bottom): ©Dan
Suzio/Photo Researchers, Inc.; p. 92: ©Tom McHugh/Photo Researchers, Inc.; p. 102:
©Jane Thomas/Visuals Unlimited.

For Katie and Danny
who share my love of books and nature

Acknowledgments

I would like to thank Dr. Gordon Cragg, chief of the Natural Products Branch at the National Cancer Institute, and Dr. Thomas Eisner at Cornell University, for their insights on medicines from nature, and my editor, Pat Culleton, for her guidance. Special thanks to my family, who graciously live through the mess of Mom writing a book.

CONTENTS

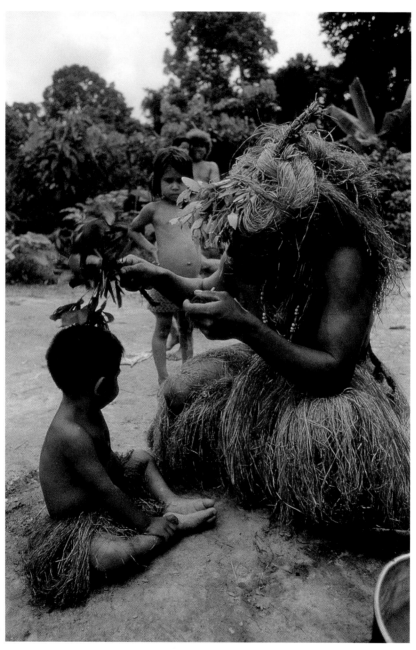

*A shaman has wide knowledge of
medicinal plants and uses them to cure the sick.*

1

SECRETS OF
THE SHAMANS

*A*s Mark Plotkin slashed his way through the dense, green Amazon rain forest, his machete blade accidentally hit a wasps' nest. A swarm of angry wasps clouded the air, stinging him many times. In pain, Plotkin turned to his companion, a shaman, a Tirio spiritual leader and healer who had been teaching Plotkin about medicinal plants. The shaman went to a bush no more than ten feet away and scraped off a small bit of bark. He crushed it in his hands and rubbed it on Plotkin's bites. In less than three minutes the pain had vanished. In five minutes, the swelling was down, and in twenty-four hours, Plotkin bore no sign of the wasp attack. When Plotkin returned to the United States after completing his fieldwork in 1982, he reported the plant's effect on the stings and discovered that it had never been studied for use as a medicine.

While Plotkin worked in the Amazon, Paul Cox, from Brigham Young University, was working halfway around the world in Samoa. He sat cross-legged on a wooden floor in a hut, listening intently and taking notes as a *taulasea*, a traditional

Samoan healer, described in detail a medicinal plant she used in healing the people in her community of yellow fever, which is caused by a type of virus. Cox hoped that the information he collected would be useful in making a drug to fight the human immunodeficiency virus (HIV), which causes AIDS.

✣ ETHNOBOTANY ✣

The scientists who are learning the secrets of the shamans are called ethnobotanists. They study the relationship between plants and people—how plants are used for housing, clothing, tools, food, and, most important, medicine. Ethnobotany is a blend of anthropological fieldwork and botany. It involves becoming a student to the healers, learning from them, and recording their knowledge about the plants they use and the way they are prepared. The scientist couples this information with botanical knowledge to identify the plants and put them through diagnostic tests called assays that determine whether a plant will have a medicinal effect on the human body.

Many ethnobotanists are medicine hunters looking for traditional remedies that may be used to make modern drugs, and they believe that focusing on the plants used by traditional healers taps into the largest laboratory in the world. It takes advantage of centuries of healing knowledge. Cox notes that "native healers have a rigorous, sophisticated methodology."[1] They know, for example, which plants are eaten by which insects or animals and how the plants affect them. If a new medicine is tried, it is tested on a dog or a pig, then on the healer. Many plants collected by the ethnobotanical approach have already passed the first hurdle in drug development: they have been proven safe and effective in humans.

One of the first ethnobotanists was Richard E. Schultes, a professor at Harvard University, who spent years during the

1940s and 1950s in the rain forests studying medicinal plants when it was not the fashionable thing to do. He has trained or inspired almost all of the ethnobotanists currently working around the world.

An ethnobotanist's job description might call for a person who is looking for adventure, who has great patience and perseverance, and who isn't particular about food or sleeping arrangements, because ethnobotanists frequently find themselves in the dense forest with only a guide to help prepare a shelter and cassava to eat. The tools of the trade include a plane ticket, a camera, good boots, a machete, and a plant press. The pay is poor, the work is hard, and the conditions are hazardous.

Ethnobotanist Jim Miller, from the Missouri Botanical Garden in St. Louis, Missouri, who works in Africa and Madagascar, once came home feeling ill and found that he was infected with five different intestinal parasites. Other ethnobotanists have suffered even worse diseases, such as typhoid and malaria. Sometimes the learning experience becomes a personal one, as Mark Plotkin found out. Not only have shamans healed his wasp stings, but he has also been the center of elaborate healing rituals for an ear infection and an injured elbow.

In the field ethnobotanists must win the confidence of the healers as well as that of local leaders and landowners so that they will be trusted and allowed to work in the area. They must be able to speak the language and understand the customs. For example, in Samoa it is important for Cox to know the arrival ceremony and to give the proper respect to the appropriate people. Often this means giving elaborate speeches and wearing a shell lei (necklace) around his neck and a hot-pink lavalava (skirt) wrapped around him. As one journalist wrote, "Skip the ethno, and you don't get the botany."[2]

Ethnobotanists focus their attention on the remote areas of the rain forest because it has been disturbed little over the centuries, so the medicinal knowledge of the plants has been honed, perfected, and passed down through generations of traditional healers. In just one culture, the Shuar of Ecuador, there are more than 250 different plants used as medicines.[3] Many of the plant species, although they are called by different names, are used by a number of cultures for similar ailments, which is a good indication that they work. For example, among the Jivaro people of the Amazon, midwives use a plant to control bleeding after childbirth. Botanists found that the plant had a fungus growing on it that turned out to contain the active ingredient in the midwives' treatment. That fungus is also used by European midwives for exactly the same purpose.

With the healer's guidance and the approval of the landowners and the government, the ethnobotanist collects about two pounds of each plant that is to be studied. An entire small plant—or the bark, leaves, and root of a tree—is called a voucher specimen. While the ethnobotanist is still in the field, the specimens are pressed to preserve them for shipping. One way is to put a voucher specimen between two sheets of newspaper. The papers are stacked and placed between two pieces of plywood and bound with straps. The bundle is then suspended a foot above a small fire. This makes the specimens ready for transport to a botanical reference library, called an herbarium.

Each page, an herbarium sheet, contains a plant labeled with the Latin name of the species, the date and location where it was collected, what the plant was used for, and by whom. While some plant chemicals remain intact in the pressed specimens for a hundred years, most compounds quickly undergo significant changes as soon as the plant is dug from the ground or the branch is snipped off the tree. In order to preserve the plant's chemical compounds some scientists store fresh specimens in an alcohol solution.

Many ethnobotanists are also called chemical prospectors, or biodiversity prospectors, because they seek out new chemical compounds and new forms of life. They work all over the world, but primarily in the rain forests, where there is the greatest number of plant species and therefore the greatest diversity in chemical compounds. They view every plant as a chemical factory. Of the 250,000 species of plants on earth, more than half grow in the rain forests, and those plants have powerful chemical toxins to protect them from some of the largest insects.[4]

Plants are at the mercy of their enemies. They cannot run and they cannot hide, so in order to survive in a world of insects and disease, plants have had to develop survival mechanisms to fend off predators and to help them propagate. They produce a wide range of chemicals as an arsenal for major chemical warfare against insects. Chemicals in the roots prevent other plants from growing nearby and taking up sunlight and valuable nutrients in the soil. Even more elaborate chemical compounds are used to attract pollinators. These chemicals are called secondary compounds because botanists believe they are not necessary for the plant's growth and reproduction. But these secondary compounds are the primary concern of pharmacologists (scientists who develop drugs) because they have the ability to heal.

Of the secondary compounds, the most powerful in terms of human medicine are the alkaloids, which are complex base compounds that have strong effects on the human body. There are over four thousand known alkaloids, and 20 percent of leafy plants contain at least one.[5] Alkaloids are most commonly found in tropical plants, but they have had a major impact on every culture. Alkaloids include stimulants such as caffeine, cocaine, heroin, and nicotine. They also include the most deadly poisons such as strychnine, potent painkillers such as codeine and morphine, and hallucinogens such as mescaline. Alkaloids often have a bitter taste, which is frequently the clue to a plant's therapeutic properties. In most cultures there are medicines known as bitters, and people tend to believe that anything that tastes bad must be good for you. The alkaloid quinine, a treatment for malaria, is one of the most bitter substances known to science and is also one of the most powerful drugs.

To understand how a medicine works in the human body, it is best to envision a chemical lock-and-key system. A specific chemical key can trigger a particular chemical reaction inside the body—such as dilating pupils or deadening pain—by fitting into a particular lock, a receptor site within human cells. For example, the key of the painkiller morphine locks into the nerve cells of the brain, blocking out the sensation of pain. When scientists are looking for a cure for a disease such as cancer, they have to know which receptor sites would shut down the cancer cell, so that they can find the right chemical key to fit the cell's chemical lock. Every year, researchers are finding more medicinal chemicals hidden inside rain forest plants.

✃ A NEW SCIENCE ✃

In the 1940s Richard E. Schultes returned from the rain forest excited by the potential new drugs he had uncovered from shamans, but no pharmaceutical company (a company that makes drugs) followed up on his leads. Seventeen years ago not one of the 250 pharmaceutical companies had a research program to study higher plants, but today more than half do. Ethnobotany is a relatively new science that has grown in popularity because American consumers spend more than $5 billion on medicines derived from plants.[6]

Science has only scratched the surface of what nature has to offer. Of all the plants in the world, it is estimated that only one half of 1 percent have been studied for their medicinal properties.[7] It is certain that the other 99.5 percent could yield much more. Most pharmaceutical companies simply screen as many substances as fast as they can, but searching every compound in every plant would be almost impossible. Scientists needed a shortcut, and they found it with the ethnobotanical approach, which targets plants that already have proven medicinal against health problems, such as fungal and parasitic diseases, which are common in rain forest areas.

Michael Balick of the New York Botanical Garden, who conducts fieldwork in Belize, reports that the plants he collects from his healer-teachers produce four times as many positive results as do random testing methods. Balick also estimates, however, that botanists have only ten to fifteen years left to collect potential medicinal plants because the rain forests are quickly disappearing.[8] Experts say that sixty thousand species— a quarter of the world's plant species—will become extinct by the year 2050.[9] Knowledge of medicinal plants will also disappear as native cultures adopt Western ideas.

≈ SHAMAN TO SHAMAN ≈

Unlike other larger pharmaceutical companies that use a mix of random testing and ethnobotany research, the small company called Shaman Pharmaceuticals, in South San Francisco, uses ethnobotany as its sole means of collecting medicinal plants. Aptly named, it tests only plants that have been documented to have medicinal use in at least three geographically distinct cultures. For a new company, it has a remarkable track record. Fewer than ten years of research have yielded a number of new compounds that have already been tested in animals and in humans for dosage and toxicity. The compounds Shaman Pharmaceuticals is developing have a head start because they have already been used by healers in the rain forest for hundreds of years, so scientists are confident they are safe for human use.

One of the healers that Shaman Pharmaceuticals has relied on is Illias Gualinga, a shaman who lives in a small village along the Bobonaza River in Ecuador. He has taught ethnobotanists much of what he knows about the remedies he uses to heal the seventy-five people who live in his small community. When Steven King, ethnobotanist and vice president of Shaman Pharmaceuticals, visited Gualinga with two other scientists, he showed Gualinga photographs of rashes, swellings, and sores associated with viral infections, yellow eyes associated with hepatitis, and foot sores common to diabetes. King asked if the shaman had patients with similar symptoms and how he treated them. Gualinga discussed a number of plants that he used, such as a fern whose roots are crushed and used as a poultice to relieve back pain. The fern is the only species of plant that grows near a tree called devil's garden. This tree exudes a powerful chemical that prevents other plants from growing near it. The fact that the fern can grow near such chemical poison means that it must have powerful chemical compounds of its own. The scientists collected samples of the fern to study.

The shaman continued to look at photographs and told King what he could treat and how he would do it. One photo showed an open sore on a foot. Gualinga described other symptoms associated with the sores, such as weak and painful legs and fungal infections. He did not see this condition often, but when he did, he boiled the bark from a certain tree and gave it to the patient as a drink. "It makes the patient very strong," he said, and he told King that if this condition were not treated, the person would die.[10] The scientists were excited but did not show it. The shaman had been describing symptoms associated with diabetes, a disease that afflicts many Americans.

Another plant growing in Gualinga's garden is used frequently for headaches, but he warned the scientists that it could also cause visions. The ethnobotanists knew that the Food and Drug Administration (FDA) would not readily approve of a drug with hallucinogenic side effects, but they collected the white flowers and enormous elephant-ear-shaped leaves anyway. Hundreds of pounds of bark, leaves, and fruits were flown to the United States for analysis, but the most important information had already been learned.

One of the compounds that Shaman Pharmaceuticals has developed is SP 303. It is based on a commonly used salve known in the Amazon as *sangre de drago*, Spanish for "blood of the dragon." The earliest European reference to *sangre de drago* was in writings by the Spanish explorer P. Bernabe Cobo, in the 1600s. It is the sap from a fast-growing tree called croton, which grows in patches of sunlight in the rain forest. The tree's leaves are heart shaped, lime green, and the size of dinner plates. A slice in the gray, mottled bark oozes a dark red sap, which native people swab onto sores and cuts. Shaman Pharmaceuticals has analyzed the sap and learned that it helps to transport fibroblasts to a wound to speed healing. A fibroblast is a type of cell that gives rise to connective tissue during normal growing or to repair wounded skin, bone, and muscle. Two products based on SP 303 from the croton tree are now being developed—one that fights the herpes virus and one to treat diarrhea.

Shaman Pharmaceuticals estimates that of the 750 to 1,000 plants that are initially looked at each year, half meet the criteria for further research.[11] Although only one or two of these compounds may go through the process of becoming a commercial drug, all of them are still a vital part of health care in native communities. The World Health Organization (WHO) estimates that plants are still the primary source of medicines for more than 80 percent of the world's population.[12]

Ethnobotanists working with a pharmaceutical company can target their research by focusing on the kinds of medicines the pharmaceutical company is looking for. For example, if a company is looking for drugs that can fight HIV, Paul Cox and others can look for medicines used by a healer to cure other viral diseases. As Cox puts it, "they [the drug companies] come up with the targets, and I hand them the arrows."[13] Some of the "arrows" that have been found by ethnobotanical research are aspirin, vomit-inducing ipecac, the tranquilizer reserpine, and the cancer drugs vincristine and vinblastine.

❧ THE VINCA DRUGS ❧

The rosy periwinkle with the Latin name *Vinca rosea* is a delicate flower with glossy green leaves. It grows wild on the island of Madagascar and in other tropical countries, and has been used as a mouthwash and eyewash, to relieve stings, and to stop bleeding. Scientists at the University of West Ontario and at Eli Lilly and Company were even more interested in the reports that in Jamaica and the Philippines, the periwinkle was made into a tea to treat diabetes. They thought that a plant used so widely must have some medicinal qualities.

Chemical studies showed that the periwinkle was not effective in fighting diabetes, but it was deadly to cancer cells. In fact, the plant had more than seventy different alkaloids, six of which killed tumors. The University of West Ontario produced a cancer drug called vinblastine, and Eli Lilly and Company produced vincristine. Both are used to treat Hodgkin's disease and childhood leukemia. Prior to their discovery, 80 percent of children with leukemia died, but with the vinca drugs, 80 percent now survive.[14]

A Hope for AIDS Patients

If scientists can find a cancer drug in a flower, then perhaps they will uncover a treatment for AIDS in a rain forest plant. In 1984 on the island of Upolu in Samoa, Paul Cox spoke to an aging healer named Epenesa, who told him of a plant used to treat yellow fever. The plant, *Homalanthus nutans*, was collected and sent to the National Cancer Institute (NCI) for testing, and it showed strong activity against HIV in a test tube. The active ingredient turned out to be prostratin, a known compound that had not been researched for this purpose before. Prostratin is a type of chemical that causes tumors to grow, so the NCI was reluctant to test it further. Cox insisted that if the compound had promoted the growth of tumors, the Samoan healers would not have used it. Since it was a widely prescribed plant, it must be safe. He was convincing, and the NCI tested prostratin by injecting it into mice. Although it did activate an enzyme that usually causes cancer cells to multiply, it did not produce any new tumors. Prostratin is not an AIDS drug yet, but Paul Cox is actively pursuing further research on this unique compound.

The discovery of prostratin's possible anti-AIDS abilities opened the door for more rain forest research. AIDS is a disease new to the human species, and traditional healers have not had to treat it. Life in the tropics is filled with many other diseases that thrive on the moist heat, however, and for these diseases, traditional healers have an assortment of treatments. One of them may be the key to stopping the killer virus that causes AIDS.

Attitudes are changing. New drugs are in such demand that scientists and pharmaceutical companies are willing to look past the superstitions, the nonscientific beliefs about illness that a culture may hold, to the hard-won medicinal knowledge native people have. After all, using plants as medicine is nothing new.

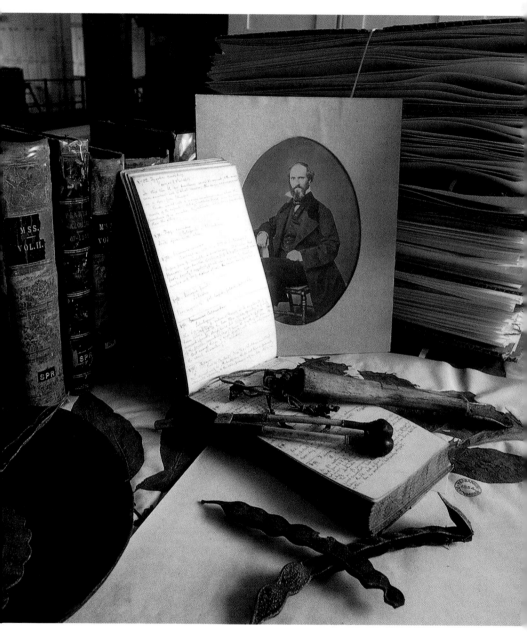

*This display shows an early record of treatments for various
medical problems and some of the dried herbs commonly used.*

2

GREEN MEDICINE

People tend to think of medicines as either natural or man-made. Natural medicines, also called herbals or botanicals, come directly from the plant, while a pharmaceutical—a man-made drug—is put together from the active ingredient's chemical parts. Although they are viewed as separate entities, they are really quite similar, because all medicines are simply chemical compounds that act in a specific way in the human body. The fact that more than 25 percent of all the prescriptions filled today were originally derived from plants attests to the long shared history of pharmaceuticals and herbals.[1]

THE ANCIENT ART OF HEALING

The earliest known written records of medicines were inscribed on six-thousand-year-old clay tablets written by the Sumerians, who lived on the banks of the Tigris and Euphrates Rivers, in what is now Iraq.[2] These tablets recorded the use of many medicinal plants, including opium poppy, licorice, thyme, and mustard. This list was later lengthened by the Babylonians, who added saffron, coriander, cinnamon, and garlic.

In 1500 B.C., an Egyptian text called the Ebers Papyrus was written. This papyrus contains more than eight hundred herbal recipes and lists seven hundred drugs, including aloe, wormwood, henbane, and castor oil. One recipe instructs the patient to put mud or moldy bread on sores to stop infection—the first hint of penicillin.[3] Another ancient text from China describes medicinal plants used more than 4,700 years ago. However, healing surely must have existed before the written word.

An archaeological site called Shanidar Cave, in Iraq, may provide some evidence for the existence of herbal healing more than sixty thousand years ago.[4] A burial inside the cave revealed a Neandertal skeleton that had been covered with a profusion of wildflowers. The hard, almost indestructible pollen of the plants survived. Under a microscope, pollen can be identified and matched to plant pollen that still exists.

What botanists found was pollen from plants that are all used as medicines today. Some of the pollen came from yarrow, a tall plant with feathery fernlike leaves and small white flowers. It is known throughout Europe as a "heal-all" plant and is still used in Iraq as a poultice for healing wounds. The marshmallow is used as a poultice for bruises and muscle aches, and as a soothing gargle for sore throats. A fast-growing weed called groundsel, also found with the burial, is used to treat stomach complaints.

Were these plants, which are still folk medicines today, used to treat the Neandertal before he died? Although we will never know, it seems logical to assume that early humans attempted to heal themselves with the very plants that provided them with food, shelter, weapons, and tools.

Every culture had its own beliefs about the causes of illness and how to treat them. Many believed in a spirit world, and that a disruption of the spirits would result in sickness. For example, a Chinese myth describes how three demons cause the disease we now call malaria. One demon carries a hammer that pounds out the headaches, another demon carries a bucket of icy water to cause the chills, and a third demon carries a stove that creates the fever. In many cultures healers were spiritual leaders as well as medicine men or women, and healing took place when elaborate and unusual rituals, centered around potent plants, were performed to soothe the spirits.

The Cherokee have a myth that tells how healing herbs came to be. Humans had killed many animals to feed their growing population, and the animals, fearing for their survival, let loose a host of diseases upon them. Plants took pity on the people, and each tree, flower, and bush agreed to provide a cure for a particular disease. It is said that when a healer doesn't know which medicine to use, the spirit of the right plant will tell him. This was, and in some parts of the world still is, a common belief.

Ancient healers were more botanists than anything else. They knew plants, and through a process of trial and error, they added different plants to their repertoire. A plant might be chosen because of its appearance—its color and shape—or its odor. For example, the liver-shaped leaves of the hepatica plant were used to treat jaundice, a liver ailment. Red plants might have been used to treat blood disorders, or heart-shaped leaves used for heart complaints. People believed that every plant was created to treat a particular illness, and the appearance or behavior of the plant was a clue to what the plant would heal. The Greeks called this the doctrine of signatures. People in each culture around the world learned which plants native to their region relieved pain, killed parasites, eased labor, or stopped bleeding. Those that worked were passed down to the next generation to be part of the culture's materia medica, all the plants that heal.

When people moved, they took their knowledge and healing plants with them. New medicines were eagerly sought out and shared, and the most effective ones were adopted by different cultures throughout the world. For instance, throughout Europe people knew the painkilling power of willow bark, and for more than two thousand years, willow bark's active ingredient was used to relieve headaches. It is still used today—the active ingredient, salicylic acid, is the basis for aspirin.

Throughout history, medicine was mixed with magic and mysticism. How else could the power of plants be explained when the causes of illness were just as mysterious? The Romans believed in witchcraft medicine, an idea that carried right through to the Middle Ages. By the fifteenth century, however, the Christian church had come to disapprove of the pagan ideas, and the old Roman herbal treatments were used only in secret. Afraid of persecution, people no longer collected plants during the day but rather under the light of the full moon, which added to their magical importance.

Some recipes clearly did not work, such as one that instructed a person with a nosebleed to hang a dried toad around his or her neck, but others were powerful medicines, and scientists are now learning just how strong the ingredients were. Henbane, for example, is considered a deadly poison; if it is ingested, it can cause blurred vision, convulsions, and even death. But a healer who knew of the plant's toxicity could safely use it in tiny amounts as a poultice for rheumatism. Today its active ingredients are used by doctors as a muscle relaxant, and to dilate the pupils of the eye.

Not just traditional healers used plants to cure. Mothers and wives treated common illnesses every day, using the cooking and healing herbs that grew in their gardens—the same types of plants that were described on clay tablets thousands of years before. With such a rich history, it is no wonder that the art of herbal healing is so strong today. In many parts of the world, herbals are still the only kinds of medicines used, and it is estimated that in the United States as many as one in three Americans now use some form of herbal remedy.[5]

✺ HERBAL HEALING TODAY ✺

If you look hard enough, you can still find traditional herbalists who will diagnose and treat patients with herbal remedies and specialized diets. Trained practitioners in many alternative therapies, such as homeopathy and naturopathy, also rely heavily on plant medicines in their practices. Most people buy their own natural medicines from a health food store, pharmacy, or grocery store, and take them as supplements much as they would take a vitamin with orange juice at breakfast.

Herbals take the place of over-the-counter medications because, for the most part, they are mild and have few side effects. Some herbs are used to treat minor ailments, and tonics are available that fortify the body with plenty of vitamins and minerals.

It is an almost impossible task to discuss the whole field of herbal medicine because there are hundreds of medicinal plants used today. Saint-John's-wort, saw palmetto, mint, and juniper grow wild in this country, but exotic plants like ginkgo, jujube, ginger, and echinacea were brought from Asia, parts of Africa, and Europe. Although herbs have been used for centuries, it has only been in the last twenty years that they have been seriously studied by scientists for their effectiveness. Ginger, garlic, and ginseng are perhaps the three most thoroughly investigated herbs.

Ginger has been put to the test many times, because it is one of the oldest herbs and most widely used for upset stomachs. The rhizome (root) of the ginger plant produces several volatile oils as well as other chemicals that are reported to stimulate blood flow, enhance digestion of fat and proteins, and stop inflammation. In one study, some volunteers were given gingerroot and then spun in a special chair. The results indicated that those who took the fresh ginger were less affected by motion sickness than were those treated with commonly used prescription medications.[6] Unlike antinausea drugs that can cause drowsiness, dry mouth, nervousness, or heart palpitations, ginger has minimal side effects, so it is used to help ease nausea associated with chemotherapy.

Ginger has other potential benefits as well. Tests show that it lowers the level of thromboxane, a chemical in our bodies that promotes clotting and inflammation; therefore, scientists think ginger might provide some protection against heart attacks, and it may be useful in treating arthritis.[7]

Garlic was used by Roman armies to dress wounds and fight infection—and for good reason. Studies show that garlic has antibiotic properties as well as the ability to fight fungal infections, and at least twenty-eight studies have found garlic effective for lowering cholesterol levels. In one German experiment, volunteers taking an 800-mg garlic tablet saw their cholesterol levels drop an average of 12 percent over four months.[8] Compounds in garlic dilate the blood vessels and may help high blood pressure, congenital heart disease, and lung conditions. Can garlic also prevent cancer? Some scientists are finding out. Preliminary studies show that garlic extracts, when put into test tubes with various cancer cells, prevent the cells from growing. They also shut down human cancer cells transplanted into mice.[9]

Feverfew is another herb that appears to be living up to its claims. It is used by people who suffer from migraine headaches, a condition for which many cannot find relief. In one study of seventy-two patients, those who took feverfew for four months had a dramatic decrease in migraines compared to the patients who took a placebo. Other herbals that have had good test results are chamomile for indigestion, saw palmetto for prostate problems, and valerian for sleeplessness. These studies are supplying badly needed scientific evidence to support what professional herbalists have known for a long time: for certain ailments, natural herbs straight from the plant work.

Some remedies are difficult to test in the lab. They are the tonics, or immune boosters, that are said to strengthen the body's natural defenses. These preparations do not fight a particular illness, but make the body stronger and better prepared to fight bacteria and viruses. The fact that they are hard to pin down adds to modern medicine's long-held skepticism about the effectiveness of natural remedies, but herbalists are quick to defend immune-boosting tonics by pointing to the hundreds and, in some cases, thousands of years of use.

Ginseng, perhaps the best-known tonic, is very popular in the United States as well as in Asia, where it originated. It is used to restore strength and vigor, increase stamina, improve digestion, as an aphrodisiac, and as a cure for many ills. Although animal studies support some of these claims, few human studies provide good evidence of its effectiveness. Recent theories suggest that ginseng may be more effective for people over sixty years old. Still, there are millions of people who take it every day and attest to its healing powers. Experiments have isolated several interesting compounds, including one that acts to suppress pain and two that may improve memory.[10]

In Germany, where herbs are commonly used, testing is done more readily, and one immune booster called echinacea, from the purple coneflower, showed promising results. It appears that echinacea reduces the severity of cold and flu symptoms, and it is believed that it increases the production of white blood cells that can destroy bacteria and viruses.[11]

❧ HERBALS AND MODERN MEDICINE ❧

Although there are many similarities between manufactured drugs and natural preparations, there are differences, too. A manufactured drug usually contains only one isolated active ingredient, whereas an herbal contains many compounds working together. This process is called synergy, and it means that the other chemical compounds in the plant work with, and enhance, the active ingredient. Herbalists feel that if you take away the other plant compounds, the active ingredient is somehow less effective.

The herbal tradition is also based on the principle of preventive medicine: plants are used to build up the body to maintain health and to enable the body to fight back when a person is sick. In contrast, modern medicine's goal is to cure a specific ill. Its medicines are like bullets designed to target certain symptoms and then to act on them.

Another difference is in the way herbals and modern medicines are treated by the United States government and the medical profession. In Europe, and in other countries around the world, natural healing and modern medicine go hand in hand, but this is not so in the United States. Very few doctors would recommend an herbal remedy over a prescription medication, in part because herbal preparations are not regulated by the FDA. According to the United States Congress, herbals come under the heading of dietary and nutritional supplements, which means that the guidelines that govern their manufacture and sale are different from those that govern modern medicines. Herbals go to market with little or no prior testing, and are manufactured under standards that some consider to be looser than those used in the manufacture of pharmaceuticals.

Pharmaceuticals, on the other hand, undergo ten to twenty years of testing, beginning with preclinical trials on animals, followed by three levels of clinical trials in humans. The results are then given to the FDA to review. Once a drug is approved, the manufacturing company receives a patent that gives it exclusive rights to sell that drug for a specified period of time. This allows the company to recoup the money spent on testing. Herbs would not fit in this system because a company could never hold a patent on a plant that everyone could grow in their gardens.

Because the herbs are not classified as drugs, companies that manufacture them are not allowed to put therapeutic claims on the labels, but the label can say how the product will affect the body's structure or function. For example, saw palmetto marketers cannot say that it will cure an enlarged prostate, but the label can say "for the prostate."

To get health information out to the public, herbal manufacturers advertise in magazines, on television, and with in-store pamphlets. A confusing set of regulations allows products on the market, but these regulations don't guarantee safety. Information is available about dosage, but not about benefits or risks. Unfortunately, it is most confusing for the consumer.

As the herbal market has grown, so have the problems. In some instances, low-quality or fraudulent preparations were made. Pills have been sold that have little or no active ingredients in them, while other products contain active ingredients that vary from capsule to capsule, and brand to brand. For example, *Consumer Reports* sampled ten brands of ginseng and found a wide variation in potency. Some pills had ten to twenty times more ginseng than others, and some had almost none at all.[12]

Herbal experts say that people should do their homework and use herbals with the same caution that they would use in taking an over-the-counter medication. Supporters of herbal regulations believe that problems such as poor quality, improper dosage, or drug interaction would be alleviated with stricter monitoring. It would also prevent the improper use of more harmful herbs such as ma huang, the active ingredient in the controversial diet aid Herbal Ecstacy and other similar products.

Ma huang is another ancient Chinese herb that has been taken for centuries as a tonic, and it came on the market in the United States promoted as a natural food supplement and advertised as a risk-free natural high. Unfortunately, that is not what more than four hundred people found out; they reported to the FDA adverse side effects, such as dizziness, heart attacks, and strokes.[13] The most troubling have been the fifteen deaths associated with the herb. Ma haung contains ephedra, which acts on the body like methamphetamine, or speed. High doses can cause a drop in blood pressure, irregular heartbeat, and seizures. Experts say that a safe dose is only 30 milligrams; however, it was being sold in doses as high as 100 milligrams. Many states have now banned its sale.[14]

The case of ma huang prompted a move to change the regulations to better protect the consumer. There is disagreement on how to do it, but most people in the industry seem to believe that there is a need for a system that recognizes the importance of herbals in health care, requires more responsibility from herbal manufacturers, and uses reasonable regulations to test effectiveness and monitor safety. The blending of herbal medicine and modern medical practices may take a while to accomplish, however; after all, the division between the two developed slowly, over a long period of time.

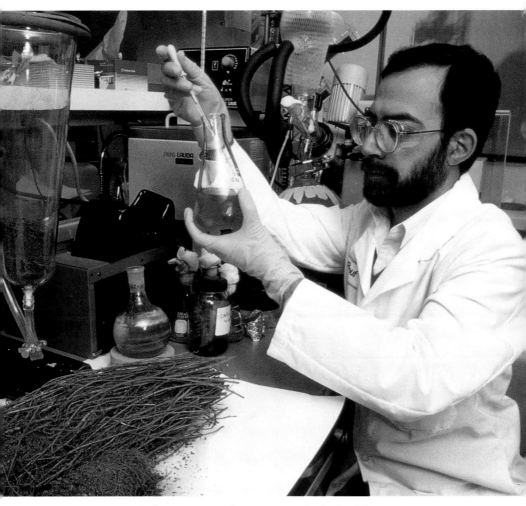

*Laboratory research on compounds obtained from
nature is an important step in the development of medicines.
Eventually, effective natural compounds may be synthesized.*

3

FAR-OUT FLORA IN MAINSTREAM MEDICINE

*T*he different paths that plant-based medicines took, namely herbals and man-made drugs, separated as the science of medicine grew, leaving some herbal remedies strictly in the hands of traditional healers, and other plant-based medicines to be dissected by scientists and made into modern drugs. Early seventeenth- and eighteenth-century scientists made great strides in learning how disease happened and how healing plants worked. For the first time, germs were seen under the microscope, and the first of many drug discoveries came from the most commonly used plants.

A classic example is the foxglove, a flower that grows in gardens all over Europe and the United States. Although it had been used for centuries by traditional healers, it moved from folk remedy to a doctors' medicine only in 1785. William Withering, an English doctor, first learned of foxglove when he told the family of a patient that the man did not have long to live. Withering later learned that his patient was doing fine after the man had visited an old woman in Shropshire who apparently attended to villagers who could not be treated by their doctors. She gave the man a mixture of boiled-down foxglove that grew in her garden. Impressed with the man's recovery, Withering began experimenting with the plant. He learned that foxglove contained digitalis, a chemical that was a powerful poison as likely to kill a patient as to save a life. After ten years of experimentation, Withering published the proper dosage, and today digitalis keeps millions of hearts beating properly by strengthening contractions and allowing the heart to rest between beats.[1]

Other drug discoveries were made from common herbs, and still others were sought out in faraway places. The scientific interest in plant medicines grew out of an age of exploration when medicinal plants were "discovered," just as Christopher Columbus "discovered" America. Native Americans had their own healing herbs such as tobacco, American ginseng, goldenseal, witch hazel, and mayapple.

✆ A CURE FROM THE FEVER TREE ✆

The first European explorers and missionaries to the New World "discovered" medicines that could treat illnesses that no European medicines had been able to treat. One of the most important was quinine, which is used to treat malaria, the reigning killer among infectious diseases in early history. A person bitten by a malaria-carrying mosquito becomes infected with the protozoan plasmodium and soon develops muscle soreness and backache, followed by chills that cause the body to shake and teeth to chatter. Then come vomiting, burning delirium, and an unquenchable thirst. When the fever breaks, the person is exhausted and depressed. That is not the end; for some people, the cycle repeats every three or four days, and for some unlucky victims, it comes every day until they die. At one time or another, malaria has plagued most major cities, including London, Madrid, Paris, Rome, and Washington, D.C.[2]

The connection between mosquitoes and malaria was not made until 1897, but the treatment was known thousands of years earlier by native people in South America, in what is now Peru and Ecuador. The bark of the cinchona tree was steeped in boiling water and was taken as a drink for several days.

The first report of this treatment came from Father Calancha, a missionary who worked in South America in 1633. He described a "fever tree" that grew on the eastern slopes of the Andes Mountains. "In the district of the city of Loxa grows a certain kind of large tree, which has bark like cinnamon, a little more coarse, and very bitter; which, ground to powder, is given to those who have fever, and with only this remedy, it [the fever] leaves them."[3]

Catholic missionaries who witnessed its use took the remedy to Europe, where it received little attention, although thousands of people, including royalty and military leaders, were dying from the fever. In Europe, victims of malaria were more likely to receive cures such as this one described in the 1200s: "Take the urine of the patient and mix it with some flour to make a good dough thereof, of which seventy-seven small cakes are made; proceed before sunrise to an anthill and throw the cakes therein. As soon as the insects devour the cakes the fever vanishes."[4] In spite of the ineffective treatments being used in Europe, quinine, then called Jesuit's powder, took a while to catch hold. It was the victim of many prejudices—religious, medical, and, later in the 1900s, political. Many Protestants would not touch quinine because it had been imported by the Jesuits, but when King Charles II of England was cured with it in 1678, the use of Jesuit's powder spread. If it had not been for these prejudices, quinine would have been in wide use, saving lives a hundred years sooner.

When the cinchona bark became part of the European materia medica, it was the first drug treatment for a specific disease used instead of the brews that contained dozens of ineffective ingredients. It was a therapeutic "smart bomb," seeking out and selectively destroying the malarial parasites hiding in the human bloodstream. Quinine was isolated as a drug in 1820 by two French pharmacists, Joseph Pelletier and Joseph Caventou, who worked for years on the project. Their first attempts failed, because they had used bark from the wrong tree.

There are more than fifty different kinds of cinchona trees, but only some of them contain the malaria-fighting compound. The yellow cinchona was the tree that yielded the yellow gummy substance that they named quinine, after the Peruvian name for the tree's bark, *quinquina*. Since then, thirty different alkaloids have been obtained from the bark of the cinchona. The isolation of quinine from the bark meant that the dosage could be more easily controlled, and the alkaloid by itself was less irritating to the stomach than was the whole-bark powder.

During World War II, part of both the Allied and enemy strategy was to cut off the other from sources of quinine. If this could be done, then the opposing troops would be severely weakened by malaria, and the war could be won. After quinine was synthesized, the battle over it was no longer an issue, because it could be manufactured regardless of who owned cinchona trees.

❧ SYNTHETIC DRUGS ❧

A drug that is synthesized, or synthetic, is made out of its chemical parts in a laboratory. Chemicals are like building blocks, and chemists are the builders. They put various chemical elements such as oxygen, nitrogen, and hydrogen together in a specified structure and effectively build a molecule of a drug. For example, the active ingredient in the cinchona bark was discovered to be quinine. Quinine has its own molecular configuration that can be taken apart and put back together again. The quinine molecule built in the lab is exactly the same as the quinine molecule extracted from bark. Under the microscope, it is impossible to tell the difference, and both the natural and synthetic molecules have the same effect on the human body.

One advantage of making drugs synthetically is that the molecule can be altered to change its effect. For instance, the basic molecule of aspirin, salicylic acid, had the unpleasant side effect of causing an upset stomach. The molecule was altered and called acetylsalicylic acid. This new molecule is as effective as the original but does not cause a stomachache. The discovery of synthetic chemistry opened up a whole new world for scientists, who found exciting new chemical compounds inside plants that could be used as medicines or as building blocks to make other important drugs.

≫ DART POISON ≪

The dream find of many Amazon explorers was curare, the most deadly plant used as a dart poison for hunting monkeys and birds. It kills quickly and without pain. Explorers and scientists of the nineteenth and twentieth centuries were anxious to get their hands on a poison that worked so well, because they knew that the only difference between a poison and a medicine was the dosage. Some believed curare could be another miracle medicine—for what, they did not know. The curare plant had to be found first.

The making of curare had been a guarded secret shrouded in ritual and mystery, and explorers who could not get their hands on it brought back strange tales about how it was made.

In one tale, curare was made only by the old women of the village. A woman would sit and stir the boiling poison until she died from its steam; then another old woman would take her place. Others reported that men made the curare, but if women or children were present, they would become sick and die.

A few explorers did bring back samples of the black gooey paste, but chemists could not figure out its active ingredients, because curare was made from many unknown plants, and the recipe varied from village to village. Scientists knew more about how curare killed than what it was made of. It blocks the communication between the nerves and the muscles, causing paralysis, first in the arms and legs, then in the body. Death occurs when the diaphragm, the large muscle beneath the lungs that controls breathing, is paralyzed. Breathing stops, and a person can suffocate in just a few minutes. For a smaller animal, death is almost instantaneous.

In some Amazon villages the potency of curare is measured by the number of trees a monkey is able to get to after being struck by a poison dart. A monkey that is able to jump to one tree before it dies is said to have been shot with "one-tree curare," the most potent. Two-tree curare works a bit slower, and "three-tree curare" works very slowly and is of poor quality. Other hunters test their poison on frogs, injecting them and making them hop. The frog must die within six jumps for the poison to be considered potent.

The way curare causes death was also the reason that doctors thought it could be useful. They felt that in proper dosage, it could be used to relax muscles that were stricken from diseases such as spastic paralysis, in which the arms and legs become immobile. Doctors also thought curare might be used to treat schizophrenia.

Richard Gill, an American traveler and rancher in Ecuador,

became obsessed with the search for curare after becoming paralyzed because of a fall off a horse in 1932. His physician told him that curare was a possible cure, but that no one had been successful in finding it. Gill set to the task of getting well enough to look for curare as only he could do. He had an advantage over other explorers, because he had lived in Ecuador and knew many local people, who had visited his ranch. In 1938, Gill was fit enough to lead an expedition into the Amazon, although he hobbled on two canes over flat land and had to be pulled up slopes by a rope around his waist. After many weeks of trading with various tribes, Gill was allowed to sit in on a curare ceremony.

On the first day, three types of vines were crushed and passed around the healer's head three times, then put in a pot. The bark of a fourth plant was added, and the mixture was boiled all night. On the second day, the bark and roots of two more plants were added, including one that Gill recognized. It was used to stun fish. This was boiled down to a thin honeylike consistency. It was strained and put in another pot, and then boiled again until it was a black foaming syrup. Gill brought back some of the paste, but more important, he brought back the various plants used in the recipe, including chrondrodendron, the plant that gave curare its sting.[5] Other tribes to the east used a different plant, strychnos.

In 1942, a Canadian anesthesiologist, Harold Griffith, discovered that curare was perfect for relaxing the muscles of the abdomen during surgery, and curare's purpose was found. There are two types of curare plants, and they are classified by the way they are stored. Strychnos is stored in pots and is called pot curare, and chrondrodendron is kept in tubes. Modern medicine uses tube curare to make the anesthetic d-tubocurarine, which can be found in almost every hospital around the world.

Chemists realized that if a plant could not be made directly into a medicine, perhaps its chemical parts could be used as a "feedstock" molecule to make a drug. Russell E. Marker was such a chemist. He recognized the similarity of the molecular makeup of steroids and the Mexican yam. A steroid is a solid alcohol that occurs naturally in plants and animals. Cholesterol, estrogen, progesterone, and testosterone are all steroids, but there are thousands of others. In the 1940s, scientists learned that steroids could be helpful in the treatment of various diseases. They noticed, for example, that women with severe arthritis got better during pregnancy, when they naturally had high levels of progesterone in their bodies. Unfortunately, natural steroids were difficult and expensive to get. Small amounts could be extracted from tons of adrenal glands of animals, but the cost would be prohibitive.

Marker, who was working in Mexico, believed he could make steroids from the Mexican yam called *dioscorea*, which Mexicans used like soap to clean their clothes.[6] One of its components is saponin, which acts as a cleansing agent, but Marker knew that he could use saponin in a different way, as a base chemical for making steroids. In his laboratory he produced progesterone inexpensively, and for a while the exportation of yams became big business for Mexico. Steroid manufacturing hit a peak when cortisone became an important treatment for many illnesses, including arthritis, asthma, and cancer. Syntex, the Mexican company where Marker had done most of his work, also invented the oral contraceptive that inhibited ovulation.

Botanists and explorers uncovered several natural and important drugs from tropical plants, but pharmaceutical companies found it easier and cheaper to rely on synthetic chemistry for the bulk of their new medicines. The more they learned about medicinal compounds, the more they were convinced that these compounds could be manipulated. Once chemists learned how to isolate a substance in a plant, they could re-create it and bypass the natural product altogether. The pull away from plants as the primary source of medicines was all but complete in the 1950s, when sulfa drugs, used for treating bacterial infections, were manufactured in labs. Synthesis was an important step for the pharmaceutical industry. Drugs made from chemicals could be made "pure," with consistent quality. They could be altered to be less toxic, or more potent, but most were still based on plant compounds.

The idea that the only good, safe drug was a synthetic one quickly took hold. Pharmaceutical companies were lulled into thinking that a drug could be manufactured to cure every ill, and that a team of scientists could create unique compounds better than Mother Nature herself. That was not the case, however; the most important class of drugs that changed health care were antibiotics that were literally dug from the earth.

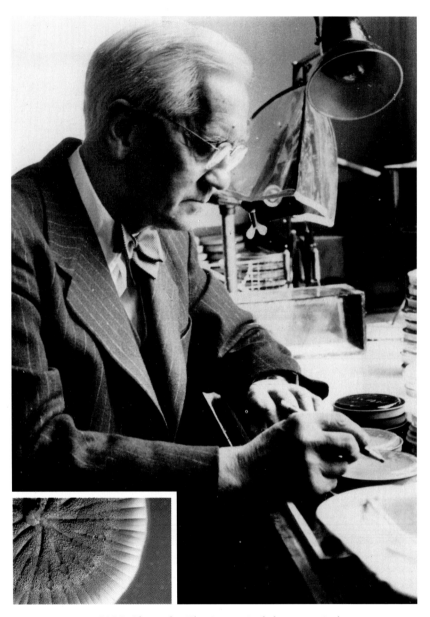

In 1928 Alexander Fleming noticed that a particular mold killed bacteria. The mold (magnified at left), which Fleming named penicillin, was developed some years later into the first safe and effective antibiotic.

4

MIRACLE MOLD

*E*very time you take a breath, you are inhaling hundreds of microscopic bacteria and mold spores. They are everywhere. Bacteria digest our food in the stomach and prevent diseases from getting past our noses, while harmful bacteria are constantly trying to get inside and make us sick. Mold spores, primitive seeds that float through the air, grow colonies of mold anywhere they land, including in the petri dishes that Alexander Fleming was using in an experiment in 1928.

Fleming was working in an inoculation lab at St. Mary's Hospital in London, England, when he first saw large yellow colonies of mold growing over a bacteria culture in a petri dish. The mold itself was not miraculous, but what it was doing was. Around the mold, there was a clear area where the bacteria had disappeared. Instead of throwing out the contaminated culture, Fleming studied it, and he found that even in diluted form, the mold killed whatever bacteria it touched. The mold Fleming was studying was not the common fuzzy green kind found on bread, but a relative that was much more rare. Fleming named it penicillin, from the Latin word *penicillus*, which means "brush," because under the microscope the mold resembled tiny brushes.

Although Fleming discovered the penicillin mold, it was Dr. Howard Florey and Dr. Ernst Chain, who, twelve years later, took up the challenge to create a usable drug.[1] They produced a pure form of penicillin and tested it on a policeman who was dying from an infected scratch inside his mouth. Penicillin was administered directly into the man's veins, but it was rapidly excreted through his urine. Since there was a limited supply of the drug, the patient's urine was collected and taken back to the lab so that the penicillin could be recycled. Florey's wife and others, who took turns bicycling back and forth with the urine, became known as the P-patrol. The man began to recover, but the recycled drug was being used up too quickly, and a month later, he died. It wasn't until penicillin saved the lives of a fourteen-year-old boy and a six-month-old baby that penicillin was called a miracle. Florey and Chain brought penicillin to the United States, where they persuaded pharmaceutical companies to mass-produce the first safe and effective antibiotic.

The discovery of antibiotics came at an important time. Infectious diseases from bacteria were the major cause of death in the United States; a patient might survive extensive surgery only to die afterward of an infection in the wound. Small outbreaks of disease could grow to epidemic proportions, as happened in 1918, when half a million Americans died from the flu.

Penicillin was such an important discovery that American soldiers were sent to collect soil samples from India, China, Africa, and South America. Employees of the United States Department of Agriculture lab in Peoria, Illinois, were instructed to collect any unusual molds as well. One employee, Mary Hunt, earned the nickname Moldy Mary because she searched through people's garbage cans and other litter. While poking through a neighbor's trash, Mary found a cantaloupe that had a pretty golden mold growing on it. When the cantaloupe mold was tested in the lab, it produced twice as much penicillin as the original mold, and this penicillin grew well in large quantities. It was named *Penicillium chrysogenum*, and it replaced Fleming's mold for use in penicillin production. Today, penicillin is not made from mold at all, but is created synthetically.

❧ MORE EARTHLY ANTIBIOTICS ❧

Pharmaceutical companies raced to find new antibiotics from new sources of mold. Bristol-Myers Pharmaceutical Company sent every one of its stockholders an envelope with instructions for collecting and returning samples of soil from their basements and backyards. Other companies contacted missionaries, oil drillers, deep-sea divers, airline pilots, and journalists, requesting that they send in samples from around the world.

In 1943, Dr. Paul Burkholder, at Yale University, sent out plastic mailing tubes to everyone he knew, and seven thousand tubes were returned with soil inside them. Of those seven thousand, four contained organisms that were active against bacteria. Further testing at the Parke Davis Company revealed that one organism found in a soil sample sent from Venezuela contained a fungus that produced chloromycetin, which killed many different kinds of bacteria, including rickettsia, a deadly bacterium that causes typhus and Rocky Mountain spotted fever.

Parke Davis started to produce chloromycetin in 1947, just when a typhus epidemic broke out in Bolivia and Peru. A doctor flew to South America with all the chloromycetin the company had. It was only enough to treat twenty-two patients, and the doctor chose the most desperately ill. One patient had been in a coma for three days, and his doctor had no hope for him. The patient was given chloromycetin, and within forty minutes he asked for a glass of water. All twenty-two patients recovered, and chloromycetin became as big a success as penicillin.[2]

Dr. Selman Waksman, who taught at Rutgers University and worked for Merck & Company, went so far as to test the mold taken from the throat of a New Jersey chicken. He found a compound that he called streptomycin, which killed the tuberculosis bacillus—something penicillin could not do. Another antibiotic, aureomycin, was discovered by Dr. Benjamin Duggar, a retired botany professor who received soil samples from friends at universities around the country. In sample number 67 from Columbia, Missouri, there was an unknown fungus he called *Actinomycetes* A-377. It did not seem particularly active against bacteria, but more testing revealed that the fungus produced a chemical that killed bacteria unaffected by penicillin and streptomycin. Aureomycin also became the first antiviral drug because it killed some types of large viruses.[3]

Antibiotics were being dug out of the dirt at an amazing rate, and it seemed fitting that these miraculous drugs should be named for the earth they came from. Miamycin was named after soil in Miami, nystatin from the New York State Board of Health laboratory, and terramycin from Terre Haute, Indiana. In the years following the discovery of penicillin, more than five thousand different antibiotics were discovered, but only seventeen were commercially successful.[4]

Two antibiotics discovered recently have revolutionized organ transplants. A patient's immune system reacts to a transplanted organ as if it were a foreign invader, and sends out white blood cells to fight it. The success rate of organ transplants, needless to say, was low at first. These new antibiotics were able to protect the new organ without harming the immune system. Cyclosporine was found in a soil sample from Norway by a vacationing researcher from a Swiss pharmaceutical company, and the newest antirejection drug from a microbe, FK-506, was found in a soil sample collected by Fujisawa Pharmaceutical Company near Mount Tsukuba, Japan.

❧ MEDICINAL MUSHROOMS ❧

Looking back on the great mold discoveries, it should not be surprising that mold has become so important medicinally. Mushrooms, which are cousins of mold, have been used in healing for centuries. Some of the most powerful hallucinogens (mind-altering substances) come from mushrooms, such as the Aztec mushroom called *teonanactl*, which means "God's flesh," and fly agaric. One species of mushroom that grows in Siberia is so rare and sought-after that in the past, native peoples would recycle the mushroom, because it still produced hallucinations after having been passed through the urine of three or four people. Their ingenuity is perhaps one of the best examples of just how extensive native people's knowledge was about plants and their effects on the human body.

❧ BACTERIA FIGHT BACK ❧

With so many new antibiotics readily available, everyone believed that infectious diseases were a thing of the past. In the 1980s, the development of antibiotics was put on the back burner, and research was focused on cancer and heart disease. Then something strange began to happen:

In March 1993, 403,000 people in Milwaukee became ill, and 104 died during the largest recorded outbreak of a waterborne disease in the United States. A one-celled intestinal parasite infiltrated the city's drinking water system.[5]

In May 1993, eighty people fell sick and forty-four people

died in some Native American communities of the Southwest after coming in contact with a mysterious respiratory illness caused by a virus carried by deer mice.[6]

In June 1994, a strain of bacteria that commonly causes children's ear infections, pneumonia, and meningitis had become resistant to some of the drugs used to kill it.[7]

Similar cases have been documented all over the world. Illnesses of epidemic proportions and deaths due to strange diseases are unsettling reminders of what life was like before antibiotics. New strains of bacteria have developed resistance to the drugs that were once used to treat them. The Centers for Disease Control attributes it in part to worldwide travels.[8] Just one tiny bacterium on one airplane can infect an entire continent very rapidly. Another reason for the drug-resistant strains is changing land use, which alters animal populations. For example, Lyme disease is caused by a type of bacterium carried by deer ticks. In Lyme, Connecticut, where the disease began, trees were being cut and the deer population was skyrocketing, putting animals and humans in greater contact with each other, and the disease spread. Hospitals are also part of the problem. A hospital becomes a breeding ground for new strains of bacteria because patients are weak, their resistance to disease is low, and they can be infected easily.

The use of antibiotics creates a situation in which the fittest microorganism survives. The rare bacterium that contains a mutation in its genes that protects it against a drug is the one that survives to reproduce and thrive. It only takes one drug-resistant microbe to multiply into millions. The overuse of drugs has caused the production of superbacteria that seem to be resistant to everything. After forty years of taking antibiotics for every ailment, people have lost some of their natural immunity to fight these microbes. They rely on drugs, but often they do not take them properly.

Some bacteria have a protective outer layer called a plasmid, which is a circular ring of DNA outside the nucleus of a bacterium that resists or neutralizes an antibiotic. Scientists are finding that this plasmid can be traded or shared with other bacteria, and even with other species of bacteria. Enterococcus, which thrives in hospitals and causes gastrointestinal infections, appears to be a superbacterium. Researchers have shown that enterococcus has mutated into vancomycin-resistant enterococcus (VRE). Vancomycin is the antibiotic given as a last resort, but the new strain of bacteria not only resist it; they appear to thrive on it![9]

❧ BACK TO NATURE ❧

So where do we go from here? The push is on to find new antibiotics and to develop vaccines that can prevent bacterial infections from starting. One way to do this is by looking in unlikely places. Most research had previously focused on fungi that caused plant disease, or molds found in the soil. Abbott Pharmaceuticals is taking a different approach, however. This company is searching out a class of fungi that lives benignly inside healthy plants and plant-eating animals. To do this, it has gone into partnership with the Milwaukee County Zoo and the Chicago Botanic Garden. The Botanic Garden supplies Abbott with clippings of plants taken from as far away as South Korea, Japan, and Siberia. The Milwaukee Zoo supplies animal dung from the American elk, Dall sheep from Alaska, and the African elephant. In the dung, scientists hope to find a new species of fungi that originally came from plants eaten in the animal's native habitat. Scientists hope that those animals born in captivity have acquired the fungus from their parents. So far, one new antibiotic has been found by looking into animals' innards: squalamine was discovered inside the dogfish shark.

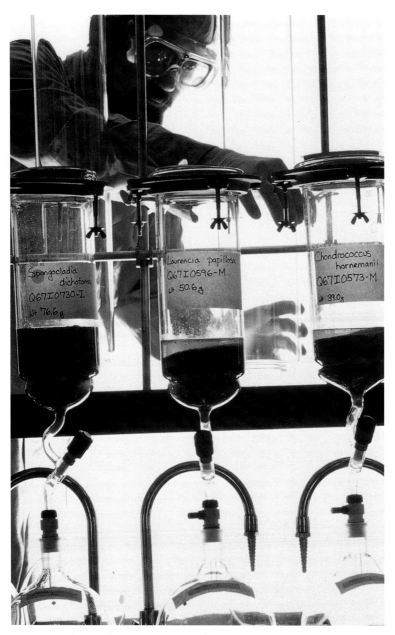

*Plant and sea creature samples are collected worldwide
and sent to the National Cancer Institute's repository.
Here extracts are tested for effectiveness against cancer and AIDS.*

5

THE GRIND 'EM AND
FIND 'EM SCIENTISTS

*T*he next AIDS or cancer drug may be an unassuming frost-encrusted lump sitting in frozen darkness at the National Cancer Institute's (NCI) Natural Products Repository (NPR) at Fort Dietrick, Maryland. It may be within the scientists' grasp, but it has yet to be discovered. The repository is the world's warehouse of medical promise, because it contains more than 35,000 plant samples of up to 10,000 different species, and 6,000 marine animals.[1] Together with microscopic organisms, the repository has 500,000 vials of extracts waiting to be tested to see which ones can kill cancer cells and the AIDS virus.

The NCI's current program, which began in 1986, is based on its original efforts in the 1960s and 1970s. For twenty-two years, the NCI's scientists tested whatever plant specimens they could get their hands on; then, the program floundered because there wasn't enough success to warrant continued research. The NCI and the pharmaceutical companies fell back on the reliable and predictable synthetic source of drug development.

One reason for the low success rate at the NCI prior to 1986 was that it was not known how cancer worked or how to screen for potential cancer drugs. At that time, there was only one kind of assay to test for cancer-reactive compounds. The common belief was that one cancer was exactly like another, regardless of where it occurred in the body. It was also believed that a drug that worked against one cancer would work against all cancers. With this kind of thinking, only a handful of compounds were developed, most of which were synthetic, and all worked the same way: by interfering with the DNA of cancer cells.

Further research on how cancer worked showed that one kind of cancer was not exactly like another, and that a compound that killed leukemia, for example, did not necessarily kill lung or skin cancer. Once new tests were developed, the NCI reopened its natural product collection program and began testing with a series of human cancer cell assays that included seven major types of cancers—lung, skin, kidney, ovary, brain, blood, and colon. In 1988 they also started to test natural compounds against AIDS.

❧ BIODIVERSITY PROSPECTING ❧

The NCI's goal is to test every species on earth, for even the most unlikely-looking species can become a winner in the pharmaceutical game. In order to do this, three organizations were contracted to gather natural products. The Missouri Botanical Garden was assigned to collect plant samples in Africa and Madagascar, plants from Central and South America are collected by the New York Botanical Garden, and the University of Illinois in Chicago collects samples in Southeast Asia. In addition, the NCI receives marine animals collected by the Coral Reef Research Foundation, and specimens from various scientists all over the world. Hundreds of botanists and biologists send their samples to the repository every year.

The NCI is always on the lookout for a new source of drugs. They have even performed rescue missions to save what information they can from threatened environments. When Hurricane Andrew devastated southern Florida in 1992, it left much of the plant life uprooted and ruined. It was a tragic sight, but even more so was the Fairchild Tropical Garden in Miami, the home of the world's largest collection of palms and palmlike relatives called cycads. Some of the species were quite rare. Before the hurricane hit, there were more than 700 species of palms and 150 species of cycads, but the storm destroyed almost 70 percent of both.[2]

Michael Balick recognized that the tragedy was also a "priceless opportunity" to collect palms from around the world, and he asked the NCI if it would be interested in testing the specimens. Officials at the NCI said yes. It would be easier, too, to clip samples from felled trees, rather than hiking into dense forests and precariously climbing towering trunks to reach a palm's lowest branches. Samples from twenty-five different palms were shipped to the Institute for testing, and although the plants themselves could not be saved, perhaps we will learn that one of them contains life-saving chemicals.

❧ GRINDING AND FINDING ❧

When a voucher specimen is clipped or captured, it is given an identification number in the form of a bar code label. Five voucher specimens of each sample are prepared. One is donated to the national herbarium of the country where it was collected, and another goes to the botany department at the Smithsonian Institution. The others arrive at the repository and are placed in one of twenty-eight freezers, each of which stands two stories high. Each freezer is filled with many racks of boxes and bags of specimens, frozen to a chilly −20°C for at least forty-eight hours to kill off any unwanted parasites or diseases. The freezers also contain vials of extracts that have already been squeezed from collected samples.

The frozen specimen, which could be a blue lobster or the giant leaves of a tropical tree, is chopped up using a band saw and a machine similar to a hamburger grinder—which is why the technicians and chemists who do this work are called the "grind 'em and find 'em" scientists. The resulting green-and-brown liquid specimens are mixed with a chemical solution and water to separate the various components. The solutions are then spun in a centrifuge, evaporated, freeze-dried, and bottled. Each extract is a pure substance, which is divided among ten small vials to be sent out for testing.

Every week, the NCI performs more than three hundred tests, which are done on sixty variations of cancers in dozens of tiny wells punched into plastic sheets the size of typing paper.[3] A drop of pure cancer the color of amber is placed in each well; then a drop of plant or animal extract is added. Everything is bar coded so that the lab technicians do not know which compound is being tested. In fact, it may be years before they find out if a compound they worked with scored a hit, which is anything that slows or kills the cancer cells. These compounds are then tested on mice that have been injected with tumor-forming cancer cells.

Not all compounds react to cancer assays. Some have no effect, and some actually cause the cancers to grow. Compounds that kill everything are usually too toxic to be used as medicines, so researchers are looking for substances that fit somewhere in the middle, compounds that are selective and kill only one or two kinds of cancer while at the same time leaving healthy cells unaffected. Each compound creates a kind of fingerprint of success or failure that can be read quickly by technicians from a computer generated printout. It looks like a bar graph, with each bar representing the effectiveness of the compound on each type of cancer. A long bar line indicates that the extract killed most of the cancer cells. A shorter bar line signifies that it killed only some of the cancer cells, and no line indicates that the compound had no effect at all.

It is important to point out that a stellar result in a test tube does not indicate a cure for cancer or AIDS. It is only the first step in the right direction. The real test would be to use it in human clinical trials, which could still be many years away. The NCI has set up rigorous testing for each drug to protect people from harmful reactions, and the FDA requires all pharmaceutical companies to test their products for dosage, side effects, and potency before any medicine can be put on the market.

If a compound does well in the first steps of testing, it is broken down into its chemical parts in order to locate the one active ingredient responsible for the desired effect. First the extract is broken down into separate solutions of large and small molecules. The two solutions are tested again, and the one that still shows activity is separated further by solvents and a process called chromatography. Each solvent separates the chemicals even further by focusing on different characteristics; for instance, molecules that are soluble in water are separated from those that are not. The extract is subdivided again and again until only one compound is left. That is the compound that creates the desired effect—it kills cancer or blocks a virus.

Mass spectrometry is used to determine the exact molecular makeup of the compound. The molecules are turned into a gas, bombarded with a beam of electrons, and then exposed to a magnetic force that causes the atoms of similar elements to group together. The scientists watch this sorting-out process, and they can determine how many molecules of each element—such as carbon, oxygen, and nitrogen—are present.

To determine the molecular structure (how the molecules

are put together) nuclear magnetic resonance is used. The compound is exposed to radiation and a magnetic field. The amount of time a particle, such as a proton, takes to begin to absorb the radiation, and the way this happens, reveal how it is arranged within the molecule's structure. Finally, once the molecular structure of a compound is known, it can be tested on animals and then on humans in clinical trials, and it can be synthesized in order to make it more palatable, less likely to produce side effects, and more effective.

❧ PLANTS OF PROMISE ☙

The NCI tests about twenty thousand extracts each year, but only 2 percent show any activity against cancer, and even fewer show enough promise to be tested in humans.[4] Those that were tested and were approved by the FDA include vinblastine and vincristine from the rosy periwinkle, Taxol (paclitaxel) from the Pacific yew tree, and a cancer drug from the mayapple. More are being tested. For example, there is a tree in China, *Camptotheca acuminata*, that looks similar to the tall stately poplar trees in the United States, but it has something that poplars do not have—four promising anticancer compounds that represent a new class of anticancer drug, which means that they shut down cancer cells differently than do other drugs currently on the market. The tree was originally tested by the NCI in the 1970s, and it was found to contain these compounds: Camptothecin, which is in clinical trials to treat gastrointestinal tract cancer; Topotecan, for lung cancer; 9AC, for a variety of cancers; and CPT-11, for lung cancer.[5] In China, this tree is called the "tree of joy," and with the many patients eagerly awaiting the new drugs in clinical trials, it just may live up to its name.

Another promising drug comes from the western Australian outback, where a wildflower of the shrub species *conospermum* grows. The plant was found by the NCI scientists in a general sweep of Australia in 1981, and, as with the hundreds of other plants collected around the world, samples of its leaves, bark, and branches were sent to the NCI. *Conospermum* was in storage for eight years until 1989, when it was tested against HIV, the AIDS virus. The results were remarkable: *conospermum* killed HIV with only a small amount of the extract, 2,500 times less than what is needed to kill a human cell, which indicated that it would not be toxic.[6] The active ingredient, conocurvone, was identified, and it is being developed by an Australian company.

Even when a substance shows good results in the screening process, there is no guarantee that it will become a prescription drug. One such instance occurred when a previously unknown vine that grows in the rain forests of Cameroon was collected and tested against HIV and showed amazing results. In a test tube, it prevented HIV from killing healthy human cells. The compound, michellamine, entered preclinical testing. Unfortunately, that is where expectations fizzled. The effects were promising in a test tube, but michellamine proved to be too toxic in studies of mice, rats, dogs, and even primates. The NCI was forced to drop it from its research. However, there is still hope that a pharmaceutical company might pick up research on michellamine, modify it, and produce something less toxic.

This just shows that in chemical prospecting, exciting compounds come and go, so it seems that working at the NCI would require patience and eternal optimism. When he was asked about new leads, Dr. Gordon Cragg, chief of the Natural Products Branch of the NCI, optimistically said, "Nothing of interest yet, but who knows? It took [the cancer drug] Taxol over twenty years to develop."[7]

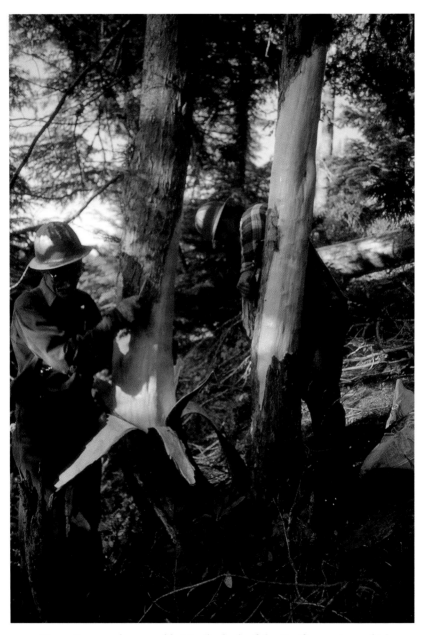

At one time, workers would strip the bark of the Pacific yew tree, which contains a compound effective against some forms of cancer. Now there are other sources of the compound, so the Pacific yew is safe from destruction.

6

TRASH TO
TREASURE TREE

*I*n 1962, USDA botanist Arthur Barclay wandered through the Oregon forest, tired at the end of the day. In front of him was a small twisted tree that he had heard was once used as an anti-inflammatory medicine by Native Americans. It didn't matter; he needed to collect it anyway. His job that day was to collect samples from every species of plant he came across, so he cut off some bark, clipped off some needles and berries, dug up some roots, put them in bags, labeled them, and moved on. So began the story of the Pacific yew tree as a cancer medicine.

For a tree that thrives only in the understory of ancient, obscure, and hard-to-reach Northwest forests, the Pacific yew tree has a long family history. In Europe, the yew was routinely planted in cemeteries because it had always been a symbol of death, and its wood was made into longbows because it was strong, flexible, and thought to be more deadly. The oldest wooden weapon ever found was a twenty-thousand-year-old spear made of yew, and the Iceman, a five-thousand-year-old body found frozen in the Alps, was carrying a bow made of yew wood.[1]

Early Greeks and Romans wrote of the yew's toxic effects, and Pliny the Elder (A.D. 23–79), a Roman lawyer turned naturalist, wrote that the yew was "unpleasant and fearful to look upon, as a cursed tree."[2] A yew tree planted at the southwest corner of a house was thought to protect the home from evil, although there was a risk of attracting witches as well. Shakespeare knew of its reputation and wrote in *Macbeth* of a witch's brew that contained "gall of goat, and slips of yew silvered in the moon's eclipse."[3]

The yew tree grows slowly but steadily for many centuries, and some of the trees now standing are known to be thousands of years old. The largest recorded is an amazing fifty feet in girth, and it is said to be three thousand years old.[4] Because of its age and stature, the yew became a symbol of immortality and is revered in many cultures around the world. In China, the yew is used to treat arthritis, and in India it relieves rheumatism. The Slishan people of Canada used the Pacific yew to treat tuberculosis as well as kidney and digestive tract problems, and for carving totems, tools, and weapons. The Potawatomi people crushed its needles and put them on sores, and it was used in sweat baths among the Chippewa, Iroquois, and Menominee for relief from arthritis and rheumatism. As long as humans have been alive, the yew tree has held a special place in history.

To the twentieth-century United States Forestry Service and the logging industry, however, the yew was a trash tree. Loggers had been cutting and burning yews in order to get them out of the way of useful trees, such as cedar and pine. The Forestry Service thought yews were so unimportant that it never recorded or counted them, as is customary with other trees. Occasionally, lumber companies stripped the bark and used the trunks of the trees to make fence posts or cheap veneer.

The Pacific yew tree sat virtually unnoticed until the 1960s, when the National Cancer Institute felt that it was losing a battle against cancer and sought a powerful ally—nature. From 1960 to 1981, the NCI screened 114,045 plant extracts and 16,196 animal extracts, and one of them was the Pacific yew tree from Arthur Barclay's collection bag.[5] Random screening seldom uncovers anything significant, but sometimes it reveals a well-hidden jewel in an otherwise worthless package—and so it was with the yew.

❧ DISCOVERING A NEW COMPOUND ❧

At that time, testing a compound's effectiveness meant taking an extract from the plant, placing it in a petri dish with cancer cells, and watching what happened. The yew bark extract, along with other compounds, was tested against cancer cells in a leukemia culture, and the cancer cells died almost immediately. The chemist who tested those bits of bark was Dr. Monroe Wall, at the Research Triangle Institute, in North Carolina. Wall was so impressed by the activity of the compound that he wrote to the NCI: "I would like to ask whether you could arrange to have this sample . . . receive a special priority, as I regard it as one of the most important samples we have had in a long time."[6] Nothing was done about it, however.

It took Wall and his associate, Mansukh C. Wani, more than a year to isolate the active compound in the bark. They named the molecule Taxol, after the Pacific yew tree's Latin name, *Taxus brevifolia.* Even after Taxol was isolated, the NCI did not take it very seriously. It was only one among a hundred other cancer-killing compounds. In order for serious attention to be paid, a compound has to either be more potent or less toxic than other compounds, or it must have a novel mechanism for killing cancer cells. The problem with Taxol was that no one knew exactly how it worked.

❧ A STRANGE MOLECULE ❧

In 1977, Taxol was sent to Susan Horwitz, a molecular pharmacologist at Albert Einstein College of Medicine, in New York City. She had a reputation for liking strange molecules, and Taxol fit the bill. It contains about two hundred atoms in an unusual and complex arrangement of rings and buttresses. "It is the kind of molecule that no chemist would ever sit down and think of making," Horwitz said.[7] Only Mother Nature could do it, and it took her millions of years, because according to botanists, the yew has been evolving as a distinct group for more than two hundred million years.

It was Horwitz's job to find out how Taxol affected cancer cells, and in one month she and her assistants knew that Taxol operated differently than did any other cancer drug. A cancer cell reproduces by replicating its DNA and dividing into two cells that are identical to the parent cell. Inside the nucleus of the cell, its DNA is duplicated, and the chromosomes line up along a central plate called the metaphase plate. Bundles of tubular structures called microtubules form a kind of scaffolding that pulls the two sets of chromosomes apart into the newly created daughter cells. During cell division, the microtubules are in a constant state of forming and dismantling.

Most cancer drugs, such as vincristine, vinblastine, and colchicine, stop the cells from dividing by halting the formation of the microtubules. There is no scaffolding to pull the chromosomes apart. What Horwitz saw under the microscope when Taxol was introduced to cancer cells were cells that formed microtubules but could not dismantle them. The cells were clogged with spaghetti-like strands. They could not reproduce, so they died. Taxol binds with a different protein receptor, inhibiting cell replication in a new and different way than do other drugs.

A new approach to cancer treatment is an important discovery, because in the fight against cancer, more than one treatment is usually necessary to help a patient. No drug is effective 100 percent of the time for every person. Those cancers that are not affected by one drug may be affected by another medication that attacks the cancer cells in a different way. The fact that Taxol had a novel mechanism for killing cancer meant that there was one more choice in chemotherapy. Studies show that only a small percentage of the drugs that are put on the market each year are a new alternative in drug therapy; most are copy-cat drugs, similar to others, but produced under a different name. These drugs do not move the field of medicine forward. Taxol, however, operated differently, and it offered new hope to cancer patients.

☙ Saving Patients ❧

In 1983, Taxol was tested on women to gauge the drug's dosage and toxicity. It had an astonishing response rate among the women with untreatable ovarian cancer. In one test, 30 percent of the tumors shrank noticeably.[8] Taxol was not a nice drug, however. Its side effects included nausea, vomiting, diarrhea, muscle aches, and more severe forms of neurological and cardiac toxicity. It even caused one death. Trials were suspended until researchers could find a better way to administer it. Because Taxol was not water soluble, it was mixed with cremophore, a type of castor oil. The mixture caused many allergic reactions. In later trials, after Taxol's dosage and administration were worked out, things looked better.

In 1985, one patient of Dr. William P. McGuire, at the Johns Hopkins University Medical Center, had ovarian cancer and less than a month to live. She asked to try Taxol. She was given the drug, and within ten days her tumor had responded to the treatment. In spite of the side effects, Taxol was proving effective against ovarian cancer and breast cancer. The doctors who worked with the patients kept urging the government and the NCI to continue with the trials, even when the NCI chose to fund research into other potential medicines instead of wasting time on problem-ridden Taxol.

❧ A LIMITED SUPPLY ❧

During the trials, a problem remained: how to get enough Taxol. Supplies were so sparse that few researchers were allowed to receive the drug. At one point, the supply was so low that one trial was postponed, to the horror of the women waiting to receive what the media were labeling a "miracle."

Taxol was a complex molecule that could not as yet be synthesized, which meant that the compound had to be extracted directly from the bark of the Pacific yew tree. No one knew how many yew trees there were, although there were reports that the numbers were dwindling fast. Back in the 1970s, several scientists recommended that the tree be put on the endangered species list to halt its destruction by the lumber companies, but for ten years cutting and burning continued even when Taxol tests looked so promising.

Only three hundred milligrams of Taxol were needed for a course of treatment that was given four to ten times for a woman with ovarian cancer.[9] On average, one patient received two grams, or less than a tablespoon of Taxol. Every year twelve thousand woman die of ovarian cancer, and it would take twenty-four kilograms of Taxol to treat those twelve thousand patients. But what did that mean to the supply of trees?

Thirty pounds of bark were needed to produce a gram of Taxol, which amounted to sixty pounds of bark per patient.[10] The yew tree was very thin skinned, however, with bark that was only an eighth of an inch thick. Even the best bark stripper got very little bark from one tree, which could yield at most twenty pounds. However, as the largest trees had already been harvested, the yield from the smaller trees was only five pounds. These figures indicated that roughly from three to as many as twelve trees would be needed for a single patient. The NCI estimated that twelve thousand patients would require 720,000 pounds of bark from up to 144,000 trees. Estimates ranged up into millions of pounds of bark needed every year in order to have even a minimal supply of Taxol on hand just for patients with ovarian cancer; more would be needed to treat women with breast cancer.

The NCI turned over the production of Taxol to Bristol-Myers Squibb, who in 1991 was granted exclusive rights to harvest the yew trees by the Department of Agriculture and Interior. In return, Bristol-Myers Squibb agreed to sponsor ecological research on the yew.

✂ SAVE THE TREES ✂

Taxol set off a debate that pitched good guy against good guy—medical researchers against environmentalists—each concerned about the welfare of the yew, but for different reasons. It was feared that widespread, uncontrolled felling would quickly eliminate the yew in the wild. Guidelines were set that required a tree had to be at least four inches in diameter to be cut, which for a slow-growing tree meant it was seventy to one hundred years old. With such a slow growth rate, the tree could never recover from extensive harvesting. The Native Yew Conservation Council was formed, and petitions were made by the Environmental Defense Fund and the American Cancer Society to the United States Fish and Wildlife Service to have the Pacific yew classified as a threatened species. Environmentalists were concerned not only about the yew but also about the habitat of animals, such as the endangered spotted owl, that nested in them.

Environmental groups were instrumental in getting the senseless practice of burning the yew stopped. Rules were set up by the United States Forestry Service and the Bureau of Land Management that required the bark peelers to leave some yews standing in order to preserve genetic diversity. A cut tree had to be left with a stump at least twelve inches tall, so that it had a chance to grow back. According to environmentalists, there still was too much waste, and the rules were not strict enough. Trees were still being felled, stripped of bark for Taxol, and then burned. All the foliage and branches were being wasted and not used in the extraction process, even when researchers knew that the foliage contained taxanes, chemical cousins to Taxol that could be instrumental in making a synthetic drug.

To the sagging logging industry, however, the felling of the yew was a long-needed boost. Those who stripped the bark got up to $2.50 per pound. The NCI paid extracting companies $32 per pound, and thirty pounds of dry bark yielded one gram of Taxol, making the cost of the drug as high as $960 per gram.[11] On the black market, however, bark cutters could earn decidedly more for their illegal efforts, and forest rangers patrolled the national forests searching out poachers. Even relatives of patients desperately waiting for this new drug to hit the market scoured the forests, and one man, whose mother was dying of cancer, was found roaming the halls of a lab where Taxol was being tested, in hopes of finding some.

It took sixty-eight individual steps to extract Taxol from yew bark. Once the bark was stripped, it was shipped to the extraction plant, where it was chipped and put into steel canister dryers used originally for filbert nuts. Once the bark was dried, it weighed about half its original weight and it looked like Grape-Nuts cereal. Then the bark was sent to Boulder, Colorado, where it was mixed with a solution of chemicals and water. A red extract the consistency of honey was then purified through several more steps. The Taxol gleaned from all this amounted to about three drops in a cup of water. Next, the Taxol was dried to a powder and sent to Bristol-Myers Squibb. Each operation had been analyzed and approved by the FDA, and any new method would be subject to the same constraints. Each part of the process had to be documented: the machines used, the solvents used, and even the manner in which the extraction room was cleaned.

❧ THE SEARCH FOR A NEW SOURCE ❧

In 1991, as the NCI and Bristol-Myers Squibb were peeling bark and extracting Taxol, other companies and universities entered the race to find new ways of producing Taxol more economically by using an abundant and sustainable source; this would mean using only what nature can easily replenish. Environmentalists, however, believed that this switch to a new source was not happening fast enough.

One solution that would save the trees was to synthesize the entire Taxol molecule, but the chemical was too complex to synthesize economically. It could be done, but the cost would put the drug out of the financial reach of most drug companies and patients.

The obvious choice, of course, was to look for Taxol in other yew species. The entire country was recruited for the cause. The *Saturday Evening Post* asked its readers to send in dried clippings from their yards, and the magazine received thousands of packets from all over the United States. People believed in the possibility that Taxol was growing right in their own front yards, and in fact it was. The ornamental yew, a dark green shrub with glossy needles and red berries, is used by land-scapers to hide a house's foundation. Tests on one variety revealed that it contained higher levels of Taxol than did the Pacific yew tree. Dried clippings had 0.02 percent Taxol, compared with the 0.01 percent Taxol in the Pacific yew bark.[12]

Using foliage rather than bark created a renewable source, because it did not kill the plant. An agricultural engineer from Ohio State University modified a grain combine machine into just the right height and shape to straddle a row of yews in order to trim the foliage and gather the clippings for research. The process of extracting Taxol from chopped needles was similar to the process of getting Taxol from bark. The foliage was placed in a solvent, and the Taxol molecule, which resembles a double-ended witch's broom, was leached out. Taxol was not the only drug extracted from the yew needles; a French drug company reported successful tests on its own product, taxotere, a chemical cousin of Taxol.

Not many yew species were found to contain the entire molecule of Taxol, but many species were found to contain part of the compound; even the Pacific yew's needles and twigs contained the most complex structures in the Taxol molecule. Starting with the partial molecule, the rest of the Taxol components could be synthesized, using a catalyst that could be reused many times.

Dr. Robert A. Holton, at the University of Florida, created a process of semisynthesis that extracted a compound called baccatin III from the English yew (*Taxus baccata*).[13] The process required only two pounds of foliage to make enough Taxol for one patient, a vast improvement over three dead trees per patient. However, the synthesized molecule that was created came in two mirror-image versions of each other. Only one version killed cancer, which meant that the other had to be strained out, wasting half of the product. Using semisynthetic Taxol allowed chemists to alter the Taxol molecule until they came up with a molecule that was a cancer killer without serious side effects.

❧ GROWING TAXOL ❧

Besides making synthetic Taxol, attempts were made to grow more yew trees. Lumber and forestry experts, such as the Weyerhauser Company, planted four million yew seedlings for future harvest, and scientists developed a way to grow Taxol in a laboratory by using tissue culture. Small pieces of bark were cut out and put in trays of nutrient-rich gel, where the cells grew into a mass called a callus. Cells from this callus were used to make more cultures. In several weeks, the calluses were harvested and dried, and the Taxol was extracted in huge fermentation tanks.

Perhaps the most startling discovery in all the Taxol frenzy was made in 1993 by Dr. Andrea Stierle during her postdoctoral research at Montana State University in Bozeman. She discovered a fungus growing on a yew tree in northern Montana that seemed to produce Taxol, even when it was grown separately from the tree.[14] She named the fungus *Taxomyces andreanae*. The yew tree produces Taxol to inhibit mold from causing root rot, but the *Taxomyces andreanae* mold was producing Taxol of its own. It appeared that by producing Taxol, the fungus was both helping the tree and improving its own survival over other fungi. There is no proof, but it is possible that the fungus acquired the gene for making Taxol from the tree through a natural process of gene transfer.

Stierle's discovery offered a relatively simple, environmentally sound, and inexpensive way to produce Taxol for commercial use. Fungi could be grown in large quantities in a growth medium inside enormous fermentation tanks similar to those used to make antibiotics. Although the amount of Taxol would be quite small, the growth medium could be altered, and the fungi could be manipulated to improve the output. More important, it gave scientists another avenue to explore: to seek out other rare, plant-produced drugs that could be accessible through the molds that grow on plants.

Any Taxol compound extracted from a tree, shrub, or fungus would have to go through extensive testing to win approval from the FDA, which considers Taxol taken from various sources to be different from each other until proven otherwise. This is required because of impurities that are inherent in each product. For example, an acceptable level of impurities could be 1 percent; however, impurities that are harmless in one source may be toxic in another.

In 1992, after thirty years of research and development, Taxol made from the bark of the Pacific yew tree was made an official drug when the FDA approved its use for women with advanced ovarian cancer. In 1994, the FDA cleared Taxol for the treatment of recurrent metastatic breast cancer, and a year later, semisynthetic Taxol made from the English yew (*Taxus baccata*) was approved for human use. This meant that the trees would no longer be cut down. The Taxol story is not over, however. Researchers continue to look for better ways to produce Taxol, including total synthesis and growth in a cell culture, as well as ways to make it more effective against other types of cancers. The story of Taxol highlights the relationship of pharmacology and botany, industry and environment, and it moved the pharmaceutical industry to search for other miracle cures hidden in unlikely places.

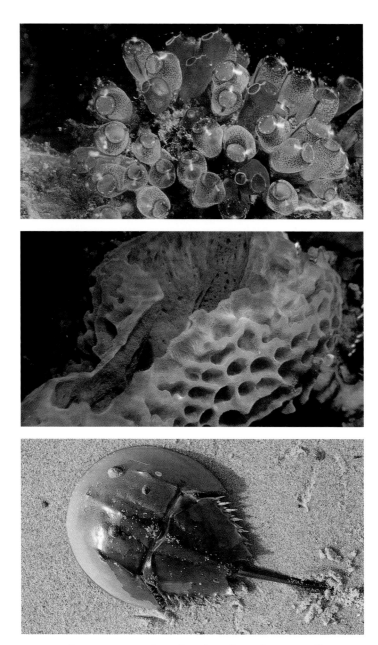

Sea creatures such as these have been the source of medicines derived from nature: sea squirts (upper), sponge (middle), and horseshoe crab (lower).

7

FISHING FOR
A CURE

A marine biology research ship rises and falls on the crest of ocean waves. Beneath the surface of the water, its crew is searching for treasure—not the shiny gold kind found in the hold of a Spanish galleon, but the slimy wriggly kind found attached to a rock at the bottom of the sea, a chemical treasure trove called a sea squirt. Its Latin name is *tunicate,* and it contains valuable chemicals that act against cancer, viruses, and tumor growth.

The sea squirt is a soft-bodied animal that looks like an underwater potato that attaches itself to pier pilings, rocks, ships' hulls, large seashells, and even to the backs of lumbering crabs. It feeds by pumping water through two large pores in its top. This odd source of future medicine was found by Dr. Kenneth Rinehart more than fifteen years ago during a five-week diving expedition funded by the National Science Foundation.[1]

On board the research ship, Rinehart extracted soluble compounds from the sea squirt and tested for any activity against bacteria cultures, fungi, and cells infected with a virus.

The sea squirt extract not only killed the virus, but killed the cells as well. The chemical that could do all this, didemnin B, is being tested and altered to improve its effectiveness while keeping its toxicity in check.

Another species of sea squirt found in the Caribbean produced a powerful chemical that is an antitumor agent 150 times more potent than the cancer drugs on the market today.[2] A fraction of a nanogram would be enough to kill tumor cells.

∂∂ SURVIVING THE SEA ∂∂

Why do these squishy, unassuming creatures have such power? Because they live in the ocean where there is danger everywhere, and they don't have hard shells, speed, or sharp teeth to protect themselves—yet they thrive.

As one researcher put it, the sea is full of soft-bodied, stationary, brightly colored creatures that are easy prey. In order to survive in this hostile environment, sea squirts and other animals developed potent toxins as their primary defense mechanism, and toxic chemicals can mean potential medicines. In the animal's body, the toxins are designed to kill outside invaders without harming the organism itself, and that is exactly what an anticancer drug is supposed to do.

Divers look specifically for soft-bodied, seemingly helpless animals that have unique responses to dangerous invasions, such as infections or venomous stings. Most often, these creatures live in warm tropical waters, where there is greater animal diversity than there is in cold water.

The sea sponge, for example, is a seemingly helpless invertebrate, but it uses a chemical called manoalide to protect itself. Manoalide regulates the sponge's chemical processes that kill intruders. Humans have a similar system. When intruders, such as bacteria, show up, the immune system sends out chemical signals telling the defense cells to activate. In humans, one of the protective processes is swelling. A wounded area swells to trap the bacteria, preventing them from spreading into the rest of the system.

The sponge, however, does not use swelling as a defense, because manoalide suppresses it. It is hoped that manoalide may be useful in humans as an anti-inflammatory to prevent the swelling associated with ulcers, headaches, rashes, arthritis, cancer, and organ transplants. The drug is so important that pharmaceutical companies have made more than three hundred different versions of manoalide for study.[3]

Other species of sea sponge have been found to contain a class of compounds, called bastadins, that interfere with the growth of leukemia cells and ovarian tumors. Another sea sponge compound disrupts cell division in tests of renal and prostate cancer. Although it is effective against cancer cells, it is so toxic that it has killed all of the lab animals exposed to it. This is where synthetic chemistry comes in—in the future, the good cancer-killing properties can be modified to reduce the toxicity.

Another way that seemingly unprotected creatures defend themselves is by using bacteria that live on the animal's skin or within its cells. The bacteria "pay" for their room and board by killing harmful viruses and bacteria, and by neutralizing venom. Istatin, a commonly used antifungal compound, was found in bacteria that protect shrimp eggs. Chinese biologist Chi-Hsin Hsu has isolated more than five thousand different bacteria, all of which are being tested for their medicinal potential.[4]

Each year, scientists take the plunge to uncover anticancer compounds from the seafloor—anti-inflammatory chemicals from seaweed, antibiotics from sea slugs, and anti-HIV compounds from algae. This is nothing new. Ancient Phoenicians were recording their use of marine life in their medical practices thousands of years ago. In the first century A.D., the Roman scholar Pliny the Elder reported that the bioluminous slime on a Mediterranean jellyfish could be rubbed on the body or taken with wine to reduce fever.

In the twentieth century, scientists believe that the same bioluminous slime might be an effective way to kill antibiotic-resistant bacteria.[5] Fish that live at the bottom of the ocean have an eerie blue glow that is caused by a protein called lumazine. Lumazine also contains an enzyme that is similar to the enzymes that make vitamin B_{12} and riboflavin in bacteria cells. By studying the lumazine enzyme, scientists can better understand the inner workings of harmful bacteria and find a way to kill them. If scientists can learn to shut down the lumazine enzyme, then theoretically they should be able to shut down the riboflavin factory inside bacteria, stopping them dead in their tracks.

Of course, a new antibiotic that works in a radically different way from those we use today is perhaps decades away, but as with all great medicines, it is a step in the right direction. Bioluminous bacteria may also be used in the future by anesthesiologists as a sensitive way to evaluate the potency and dosage of anesthetics during surgery, because bioluminous bacteria dim when they come in contact with certain drugs.

✌ Drugs From the Sea ✌

More than a decade ago, only one drug company in the United States had a marine department, but today all the major pharmaceutical companies have full-time staffs that do nothing but explore the oceans. Turning to the sea is a logical step in the search for new drugs because science has studied only 2 percent of all marine chemicals. According to NCI, 50 percent of marine microorganisms reveal new and unique compounds, whereas only 1 percent of soil specimens show anything new.[6] New screening methods allow chemists to test up to a thousand compounds a day, and assays can be done right on board the research ships. Although it costs twice as much to get a specimen from the sea as it does to get one on land, the effort seems worth it. The majority of the natural compounds that show promise as anticancer drugs come from the sea, and NCI's marine division has so far uncovered one substance from blue-green algae that is active against the AIDS virus in a test tube.

When an organism is found to have new drug possibilities, the concern then switches to conservation. Sea farms are used to grow mass quantities of disease-fighting sea organisms such as the difficult-to-raise sea sponge, which is being farmed for the first time in New Zealand. The marine chemist in effect is "growing" halichondrin, one of the six drugs currently in clinical trials. Marine microbes are also being cultivated.

One of the most difficult tasks in marine farming is finding the right growth medium. Terrestrial microbes grow well in glucose, but there is no glucose in the ocean, so scientists are experimenting with growth mediums, just as a chef fiddles with a recipe, except the marine farmer uses ingredients such as fish meal, fish oil, and crushed crab shells.

❧ MARINE VETERANS ❧

Besides being tested for chemical compounds, marine life has been instrumental in some of the major medical discoveries in history. Animals such as the starfish, shark, squid, and lobster are used as models for understanding human disease because their cellular structure is a primitive version of our own, with simple mechanisms to fight disease. Their structures are larger and easier to use in experiments. For example, the axon of a squid is a primitive version of our largest nerve, the sciatic nerve that runs down the backs of the legs, yet the squid axon is many times thicker than the human nerve and easier to manipulate. Researchers are using squid to try to understand diseases of the brain and nervous system, such as Alzheimer's and Lou Gehrig's disease.

One veteran of the medical world is the horseshoe crab, which can be found all along the eastern seaboard. This helmet-shaped crustacean has been responsible for discoveries in ophthalmology, bacteriology, and surgery. The most remarkable aspect of the horseshoe crab is its blood, which turns a rich cobalt blue when exposed to oxygen in the air.

In 1955, at the Marine Biological Laboratory in Woods Hole, Massachusetts, Dr. Fredrick Bang was conducting an experiment on the circulation of blood in a horseshoe crab when the crab's blood thickened and clotted. Although this ruined Bang's experiment, it prompted many others. Special cells—amoebocytes—in the crab's blood were found that detect bacteria and endotoxins (chemical poisons given off by bacteria). When endotoxins are present, the cells will clot. The chemical in the cells that causes them to clot was called limulus lysate. It was developed as a way to detect toxins in medicines, blood, and other fluids.

To make limulus lysate, the largest crabs, which are usually the females, are captured and taken to a lab so that some of their blood can be removed, after which the crabs are released back into the sea. The blue blood is spun in a centrifuge to separate out the amoebocyte cells from the plasma. Distilled water is added to the cells, causing them to explode, and releasing the lysate, which is then freeze-dried to a fine white powder and packaged. One quart of lumulus lysate costs $15,000, but for the job it does, it is priceless.

Prior to using lysate, doctors used rabbits to test for endotoxins, but this is not done today. If there is an infection, the lysate will clot. If there is no infection, the solution will remain the same. The test takes only fifteen minutes, and it has saved countless lives.

In 1976, there was a deadly outbreak of swine flu. The federal government initiated a widespread flu vaccination program, but some of the vaccine had become contaminated with endotoxins, and people inoculated with it died. Because of this tragedy, the FDA required that all flu vaccines be tested with lysate before being released to the public.[7] It is used to test every injectable drug and solution, as well as blood used in transfusions. It is also being studied as a possible anticancer drug. The use of horseshoe crabs does not stop there, however. The crab's shell is used to make surgical thread and bandages that can actually help wounds heal faster.

THE CONTROVERSY OVER SHARK CARTILAGE

One sea creature that caused quite a stir when it was used in cancer studies was the shark. It all began when scientists looking for a way to shut down cancer cells began to experiment with cartilage.

Scientists know that when a cancerous tumor begins to grow in the body, it must recruit a network of blood vessels that will supply the tumor cells with nutrients. In order to do this, the tumor cells send out growth factors, chemicals that stimulate the surrounding blood vessels to grow new branches toward the tumor. If this process, called angiogenesis, could be stopped, then the tumor cells would starve and die, and cancer would be cured. Scientists wondered if cartilage, which doesn't have many blood vessels, contained a chemical that prevented blood vessels from growing.

A protein was found in cow's cartilage that, when injected into lab animals, inhibited the growth of blood vessels and also stopped tumor growth. More research was conducted using sharks because a shark's skeleton is made entirely of cartilage.

One eight-foot-long shark yields three pounds of cartilage, compared to three ounces of cartilage from a cow. Also, in the twenty-one years that the Smithsonian Institution's Registry of Tumors in Lower Animals had been recording, only twelve tumors were found in sharks, which was only 1 percent of all tumors found in fish.[8] Experiments showed that in a test tube, shark cartilage also appeared to inhibit the growth of tumors.

The test results were reported in scientific journals, but the news soon hit the headlines with misleading claims that shark cartilage could cure cancer and stop AIDS. Because of the promising test-tube results, many companies quickly began profiting by selling shark cartilage powders and ointments. Thousands of people desperate for a cure took the products, hoping that the claims were true. This caused a media frenzy and a conservation scare. Once again, the quest for medicines from nature raised important environmental issues about using another living species as the raw material to manufacture drugs.

Almost immediately after the announcement that shark cartilage stopped cancer cells from growing in a test tube, there was an enormous increase in the demand for sharks, and in tropical waters, the shark became the most profit-making catch for local fishermen. Poaching and fishing for sharks outside legal fishing limits threatened their survival, because sharks don't mate until they are almost ten years old, and when they do they only have one or two offspring per breeding cycle. Sharks were being caught at a faster rate than the species could handle.

Meanwhile, new tests conducted on humans revealed disappointing results. Shark cartilage inhibited tumor cell growth in a test tube, but it did not have the same effect in the human body.[9] Sharks were being caught and made into a medicine that had not been proven to work.

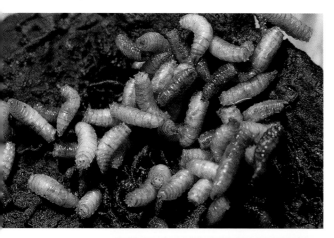

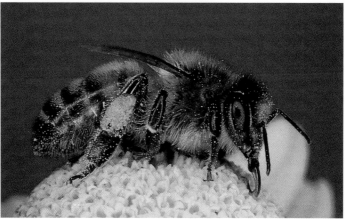

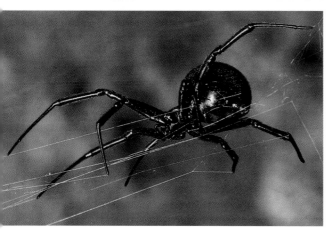

Maggots (upper) *eat dead flesh and can be used to clean out a deep wound. A bee* (middle) *produces a substance that increases the effectiveness of certain antibiotics. Spider venom, such as that from the Black Widow* (lower), *is being studied for treating nervous system disorders.*

8

CREEPY, CRAWLY CURES

With all of the scientific advances made in modern medicine, why are there doctors still using bloodthirsty leeches in operating rooms? Is it a case of malpractice or a cause for celebration? Well, if you were having a severed limb reattached, you would want these swamp suckers at your side.

That's what a U.S. Navy helicopter pilot found out when he had his fingers torn off in a freak accident. The patient waited at the hospital while twelve medicinal leeches were express-mailed in a cooler labeled "the biting edge of medicine." They would provide the postoperative help the plastic surgeon needed in order to put the pilot's fingers back in place successfully.

More than sixty-five thousand leeches are used each year in hospitals, and more than five thousand Americans owe them their gratitude for successfully replaced body parts.[1] Reattaching a finger costs approximately $20,000, but it would be a waste of time and money if not for the leeches, which cost only $7 each.[2] Leeches can do what no mechanical instrument or modern drug can do. They buy precious, flesh-saving time that allows the reattached body part to mend.

A surgeon can close a torn major artery under the microscope, but veins are more fragile and difficult to reconnect. Veins are also prone to clotting, so reattached body parts have a strong inflow of blood through the arteries into the reconnected tissue, but very bad outflow of blood through the clogged veins. This causes swelling, and without a sufficient flow of blood, the tissue will die. The leech acts like a safety valve on a steam engine. The biting and bloodsucking action of the leech relieves the built-up pressure on the tissue until new capillaries can grow and veins can carry the blood away naturally.

The leech's Latin name, *Hirudo medicinalis*, attests to its reputation as a veteran at the healing game. In the 1700s and 1800s, leeches were one of the primary tools of doctors. Unfortunately, they were also used to treat illnesses they could not cure. Leeches were put on the temples of people with headaches to relieve pressure on the brain, and they were placed on patients to relieve fever by removing "bad blood." Leeches became synonymous with quacks and charlatans, which is why leeches disappeared from the medical scene until recently, when plastic surgeons around the world realized that leeches were the perfect tool for healing severed body parts.

It is not only the leeches' bloodthirsty qualities that are attractive to doctors, but their saliva as well. When a leech bites into flesh, it cuts into the skin with three jaws full of razor-sharp teeth. It then secretes a chemical called hirudin in its saliva, which numbs the wound and prevents blood from clotting. The blood will flow freely, and the leech will suck up to a tablespoon of blood until it is full and then falls off, but another tablespoon of blood will flow before it clots.

The rare, giant, eighteen-inch-long Amazon leech produces hemetin, a different anticoagulant that not only prevents clots from forming but breaks down existing clots. Hemetin can be used effectively to stop a heart attack in progress and to limit the damage. Scientists believe that the leech is a veritable living pharmacy, and that there are more active chemicals still to be found.[3]

Saliva from a vampire bat is also being studied as a possible heart attack treatment, because it has the same ability to dissolve blood clots. When a bat bites another animal, it must lick the blood off the wound while Bat-PA, a protein in the bat's saliva, allows the blood to flow freely as long as the bat continues to lick.

❧ MAGGOT MEDICINE ❧

Leeches and vampire bats probably fit more comfortably into mainstream medicine compared to the species that entomologist David Rogers works with at Oxford University, in England. He studies green bottle houseflies and their offspring the maggot. It is the maggot that shows medicinal promise, and it may follow in the footsteps of the leech in healing wounds and fighting infection.

Civil War field doctors noticed that the patients who fared the best often were those who were not treated at all.[4] Soldiers whose wounds were deep, infected, and maggot infested were thought to be beyond medical help, but to the surprise of the physicians, these victims sometimes recovered more quickly, and in greater numbers, than the soldiers whom the doctors treated.

It turns out that maggots, which are the larvae of the fly, eat only dead and dying tissue, along with the bacteria lurking in the wound. As they feed, the larvae are actually cleaning the area, at the same time leaving healthy tissue alone. Studies show that maggots also excrete large quantities of allantoin, a substance also found in the herb comfrey, that has the ability to sterilize the tissue.

Many doctors in the United States and Canada used maggots to clean out deep wounds, and in 1934, a USDA survey showed that 91.2 percent of the doctors in the survey used and were happy with the way maggots worked.[5] Maggots fell into disfavor when antibiotics came into wide use, but in an age of increasing antibiotic-resistant bacteria, maggots may be back in business. Some researchers believe that maggots do a better job of cleaning out a wound than do antibiotics because they go right to the problem. Antibiotics, on the other hand, circulate through the body and can kill off good bacteria in the digestive tract as well as the bacteria in the infection. By using approximately ten maggots per square centimeter of open sore, doctors can effectively shrink a wound by 25 percent in one week. In one study, ten patients who were deemed untreatable by ordinary methods were completely healed within a month.[6]

There is only one problem: it is hard for patients, nurses, and doctors to get over the "yuck factor" of maggots. Patients do not like them on their skin, and nurses and doctors do not like handling them. Maggots are very effective, though, and it costs next to nothing for a hospital to raise its own supply in sterile conditions. One doctor, who was an entomologist and now works at the University of California, has been treating patients with maggots at the Veterans Affairs Medical Center for several years with great success.[7]

❧ DRUGS FROM BUGS ❧

If maggots have made it into medical books, then other bugs as sources of drugs can't be far behind. As a matter of fact, Dr. Thomas Eisner, an entomologist at Cornell University, believes that insects are the next great untapped resource for potential medicinal compounds and have been long overlooked by pharmaceutical companies.[8] There are no drugs from bugs on the market yet, but in time there may be. Perhaps it could be an antibiotic from a beetle, a sedative from a millipede, or a birth control compound from the silphid or carrion beetle.

Eisner and other entomologists, who are looking for insects that have healing properties, focus on the insects that are colorful. The brightly colored ones say, "Watch out. If you eat me, you are in for a surprise." These insects do not use camouflage for a defense. Instead they have toxins so potent that an advance warning of brilliant red or neon yellow is all that is required to ward off potential enemies.

Nocturnal insects, most of which are not brightly colored, are viewed in another way. Entomologists ask themselves, "Who eats whom?" The firefly, which signals with its mini flashlight, is not eaten by birds. Why? Eisner found out that the firefly contains a compound that is a heart stimulant. If a bird were to eat it, it might cause the bird to become sick or die. It was discovered that the firefly has antiviral properties as well.

So far, insects seem to contain the same variety of chemical compounds as plants. There are antiviral substances, antibiotics, stimulants, and depressants. In addition to their own defenses, they also take in other chemical substances from the plants they eat, so when entomologists collect insects, they also note what kind of plant it was feeding on at the time of capture. It is too early to tell for sure, but Eisner believes that insects may prove to be even more chemical rich than plants are.[9] If that is true, then entomologists will be busy for a long time, because every fourth animal in the world is an insect.

❧ ANCIENT INSECT REMEDIES ❧

Eisner sees insects as walking miniature medicine cabinets, and it appears that the ancient Egyptians thought so too, because the Ebers Papyrus contains hundreds of insect remedies. An important aspect of deciphering an insect's healing abilities was the doctrine of signatures. The way the insect looked told the healer what ailment the insect could cure. In Latin this is called *Similia similibus curantur*, which means "Like cures like." For instance, hairy insects, such as bees, were used to cure baldness. Singing insects, such as grasshoppers and crickets, were used to cure sore throats and ear problems, even though crickets and grasshoppers actually make their familiar chirping sound with their legs and wings. The earwig, so named because its wing is shaped like an ear, was mashed and mixed with the urine of a hare and put in the ear to cure deafness. Most insects are incredibly prolific, having thousands of offspring in a season, and this was seen as a sign that the insect might be good for treating infertility. For the most part, these medicines did no harm, although they seldom did good either, at least not for what they were intended.

But recent studies now show that some recipes were indeed medicinally useful. Certain insects, such as the cicada and cricket, were prescribed by ancient Roman physicians and eighteenth-century doctors as diuretics and for urinary and bladder complaints. Today, scientists know that the blood of crickets, cicadas, and other related insects contain high levels of sodium, which plays an important role in regulating water balance in the human body. In the human kidney, the concentration of sodium helps control the reabsorption of water. When Roman physicians prescribed these insects to be roasted and taken for bladder pain, they may have hit on a novel remedy in place of using salt, which at that time was a precious commodity.[10]

Insect blood is also full of many different kinds of antibiotic secretions, such as the allantoin found in the housefly maggot. The old Chinese remedy of pounding seven bedbugs, mixing them with cooked rice, and applying the paste to infected sores was probably effective for stopping the spread of infection, and it helped the wound heal faster. Similarly, a recipe from 1590 in Europe recommended removing the heads of bedbugs and placing them directly on open wounds.

Even the pesky ant was drafted in the war against disease. In the Amazon, army ants were used to close surgical wounds. Native people would close cuts by letting the sharp mandibles of the soldier ants close around the incision, effectively suturing it. The ants' bodies were then snapped off, leaving the heads with their jaws clamped shut on the wound. Carpenter ants were used for the same purpose in parts of Africa, India, and the Mediterranean.

Bees gather the sap that oozes from the buds and bark of poplars, firs, and other trees and mix it with their own secretions to form what the ancient Greeks called *propolis*, which means "before the city." It was believed that the bees coated the entrance to their hives with propolis as a way of defending themselves against intruders. If an intruder happened in, it was coated with the propolis and killed. Propolis has been used by people for centuries to boost the immune system, and in tests, antibiotics given in conjunction with propolis worked from ten to a hundred times better than antibiotics alone.[11] It has been claimed that propolis also has antibacterial and antiviral action and can lower blood fat.

✖ VALUABLE VENOM ✖

Cleopatra once experimented on prisoners to find a fast-acting poison and found that wasp venom was very effective. Since then, many experiments have been conducted with wasp and bee venom, but mostly to find a good use for the potent chemicals. The venom blocks sensory nerves, lessening the sensation of pain, and increases blood flow, which is useful in treating rheumatism, a painful condition that stops circulation. Today there are several commercial preparations of bee venom, such as Apicur, Virapin, and Forapin.

Spider venom is also a promising compound for treating nervous system disorders. It is a complex mixture of sometimes more than a hundred chemicals, but spider venom tends to be very specific in its actions, working on one particular area. The venom of a Japanese spider works to block a substance called glutamate, which is necessary for the transmission of ions through nerve cells. It is thought that glutamate plays an important role in nerve cell death in a patient who has suffered a stroke or injury to the nervous system, so spider venom just might be an effective medicine to reestablish nerves damaged by strokes.

A leap up the food chain leads chemical prospectors to *Phyllobates terribilis*, a harsh name for a tiny frog only two inches long. It is also called a poison-dart frog, and it is more deadly than other animals ten times larger. *Phyllobates terribilis*, found only in a small area of the lowland rain forest in western Columbia, is lethal to the touch. Its skin has hundreds of minute pores that secrete a poisonous sweat called batrachotoxin, which causes irreversible muscle contractions leading to heart failure. Another frog found in Ecuadorian streams excretes a chemical that deadens pain and is two hundred times more powerful than morphine.[12]

There are about 135 different species of poison-dart frogs, but only fifty-five are known to be toxic, and only three are used by traditional hunters to tip their arrows. These frogs range in size from half an inch to three inches long, yet they are not hard to see. As is true of most poisonous animals, they are brightly colored in reds, yellows, blues, and greens to warn predators to stay away. One frog, *Dendrobates auratus*, found in the forests of Toboga Island, Panama, frequently encounters tarantulas that eat other frogs the same size, but stay far away from this one. If a tarantula were to take a nibble, it would soon foam at the mouth and die. Yet to drug researchers, the pumil-iotoxin that *Dendrobates auratus* exudes may be more helpful than deadly. Researchers are hoping that someday it will be used to jump-start the human heart after a heart attack.

John Daly, of the National Institutes of Health, has studied frogs in the wild and those bred at the National Aquarium in Baltimore. He has identified almost three hundred alkaloid compounds secreted by various frogs, and has found some that are similar to cocaine, morphine, and curare.[13] Daly can judge the toxicity of the frog by taste, although he warns others not to try it. He only does this with captive frogs, which gradually lose their toxicity after being taken away from the wild. Frogs born in captivity are nontoxic, and Daly believes that a frog's toxicity may be due to its diet.

Traditional hunters in the Amazon, who use the frogs to poison their darts, taste the poison indirectly, because after killing an animal the hunter licks the carcass to find the part affected by the toxin, which will then be cut away. Making their poison darts takes some courage, too. They are made from the wood of a palm tree with fibers from the seeds of the kapok tree. To make a dart poisonous, the hunter must catch a frog, place it in a bowl, and hold it in position by putting one thumb on the frog's toe. Using a leaf as a shield at all times, the hunter rubs the dart on the back of the frog. The sweat of one frog can coat as many as fifty darts, and it will retain its potency for up to a year.

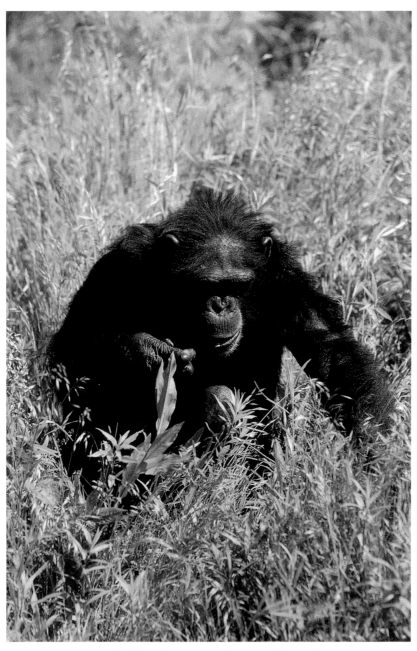

*Ethnobotonists observe the eating habits of
chimpanzees to learn how the animals use certain plants.*

9

MONKEY MEDICINE AND PHARMACEUTICAL FARMS

*C*himpanzee "CH" lay on the ground while the other chimpanzees in her troop foraged for food. The female chimp in Tanzania's Mahale Mountain National Park was obviously sick. She had no appetite, had darkened urine and bowel irregularity, and she was extremely lethargic. After several hours, "CH" slowly made her way to a shrub, *Vernonia amygdalina*, which is rarely eaten by chimpanzees. She plucked a leaf, sucked on it and swallowed the bitter juice, then spit out the leaf. The next day, "CH" was visibly better. Michael A. Huffman, of Kyoto University, in Japan, one of the primatologists who observed "CH's" behavior, later learned that people living in the Mahale area use the extracts of bark, stems, roots, seeds, and leaves of the same shrub to treat intestinal upset and appetite loss as well as scurvy, malaria, and rheumatism.[1] It appeared that "CH" knew how to make herself feel better, and laboratory tests on the plant proved that she had chosen her medicine correctly. *Vernonia amygdalina* is loaded with a bitter-tasting substance that kills harmful bacteria and intestinal parasites.

❧ A New Approach to ❧ Medicine Hunting

Are chimpanzees eating leaves to make themselves feel better? We may never really know if it is a conscious effort on their part, but it has sparked a new science called zoopharmacognosy, the study of animals and how they use medicinal plants. Scientists who follow primates around have recorded many instances of monkey medicine.

Harvard anthropologist Richard W. Wrangham watched chimpanzees in the Gombe National Forest in Tanzania as they rose one morning. Instead of going to the fruit trees for breakfast, as they had done every other morning, the chimpanzees marched twenty minutes to eat plants of the *Aspilia*, which is related to the sunflower. The chimps didn't seem to enjoy their breakfast—they wrinkled up their noses with each bite—but they continued to pluck one leaf at a time and swallow each one whole without chewing. Wrangham himself tried the leaves and admitted that they were "extremely nasty to eat."[2]

Samples of the plant were sent to biochemist Eloy Rodriguez at the University of California, Irvine, to be analyzed. The leaves contained a red oil, thiarubrine-A, which kills fungi and parasites, including the tiny worms that commonly infest chimps. Thiarubrine-A is one of the most powerful antibiotics ever discovered, and tests show that it also kills cervical cancer cells in a test tube as effectively as other cancer drugs currently used.

Rhesus monkeys at Cayo Santiago, Puerto Rico, regularly eat dirt that contains high levels of kaolin, the active ingredient in the antidiarrhea medicine Kaopectate. Muriqui monkeys in Brazil appear to reduce their fertility by eating the leaves of one plant, but they eat another plant, monkey ear, when they are ready to increase their fertility. One scientist in Costa Rica proposed the idea that primates could actually influence the sex of their offspring by eating certain plants.[3]

Primates are not the only species that seem to medicate themselves. A sixty-year-old pregnant elephant, who had a daily routine of walking five kilometers and eating a standard mix of plants along the way, suddenly altered her habit. Surprised biologists followed her for twenty-eight kilometers until she stopped and devoured an entire tree, down to its stump. The tree, *Boraginaceae*, was not known to have been eaten by elephants before.

Four days later, the elephant gave birth to a healthy baby. The story meant nothing until the researchers found out that pregnant women in Kenya used tea made from the bark and leaves of the same tree to induce labor.[4]

Black bears at the Cheyenne Mountain Zoo, in Colorado Springs, have also been observed using plants. They chew the root of the *Ligusticum porteri* plant into a mulch, and then spread it on their fur to control parasites. The same plant is well known among southwest Native American healers for being an effective insecticide, heart tonic, antibiotic, and anesthetic.

Following animals around may prove to be more beneficial for locating medicinal plants than does working with traditional healers. According to Harvard botanist Shawn Sigstedt, native cultures are losing their knowledge of medicinal plants at a rapid rate, because of the encroachment of Western ideas.[5] Animals, on the other hand, have been using the forest as a pharmacy for thousands of years and continue to do so without interruption.

However, there is one catch—extinction. Clearing forests for human use causes a loss of medicinal sources for the animals that have come to depend on them. That problem might take a backseat to an even greater threat: killing animals for their body parts to make Asian folk remedies.

❧ ASIAN ANIMAL MEDICINE ❧

For thousands of years, Asian people have relied on plant and animal folk remedies for healing, but today some of the ancient practices are threatening already endangered species. Large game animals are the most at risk.

The Siberian tiger has been hunted to near extinction, and only a few hundred remain in the wild. China, Japan, and Korea eagerly import tiger parts, including skin, whiskers, eyelashes, bones, and sexual organs to use in traditional medicines. The bones are ground up for powders, and parts are sold as aphrodisiacs, substances used to increase sexual feelings.

Conservationists are trying to place bans on tiger hunting, but the trade in tiger parts has increased since Russia opened up economic trading, and because living conditions are so harsh that the sale of one tiger for around $25,000 could support a family for an entire year.[6]

Monkey brains, rhino horns, seal penises, sea horses, and bear gall bladders are all in demand. The black rhinoceros is on the verge of extinction because its horns have been used to make a painkiller and a treatment for fever and skin ulcers since 200 B.C.[7] Although scientific studies do not support most of these claims, in some parts of the world, rhino horns are still three times more valuable than gold. Rhinos' bones are also powdered and made into pills to treat laryngitis and nosebleeds. Hong Kong, the largest producer of Asian medicines, deals with over one million pounds of pharmaceutical animal parts each year. Many conservationists are worried that this lucrative trade will cause the decrease of an already dwindling wildlife population.

❧ A Spreading Threat ❧

It is difficult to stop the practice of using animal parts for healing, because it is deeply rooted in tradition. Also, unfortunately, this ancient practice is now spilling over into European countries, Canada, and the United States. One conservationist claims that Asians want Canadian wildlife because they have destroyed their own.[8] In Canada, bears are being illegally killed every day, because poachers can get up to $5,000 for the claws, paws, and gall bladder. After these parts are removed, the rest of the bear is left in the woods to rot, while the gall bladders are dried and crushed into a powder and sold as a remedy for pain and inflammation.

To respond to the growing market, there are farms that raise certain animals to be made into traditional Asian medicines. Elk and deer are raised for their velvet, the fuzzy fur that grows on the antlers each spring. In some Asian countries, the velvet is used as an aphrodisiac. Although some say that these farms prevent the illegal taking of wild animals, others argue that it fuels the need and desire for these substances.

While some animals can be raised in captivity, the rare tiger and rhino cannot. Commercial use may be the salvation of some species, because commercially raised animals will never become extinct; however, commercially raised animals are no longer wild, and many environmentalists feel that the trade-off is too great for us to make.

❧ Down on the Farm ❧

The use of wild animals for a source of medicine is arguably a hot issue, but the use of domesticated animals that have been used for clothes, food, and labor since domestication began

97

thousands of years ago has taken a new twist. Herman, a large black-and-white bull, has made medical history: he is the first transgenic dairy bull.[9] *Transgenic* literally means "moving genes," and that is what scientists have done—moved genes from one species of animal to another. The scientists at GenPharm in Leiden, the Netherlands, were a little disappointed that the first offspring was a male, but scientists hope that when he is grown and mated, Herman will sire the first dairy cow able to produce lactoferrin, a human protein, in her milk. Lactoferrin, which is normally produced in human breast milk, contains an important antibacterial agent that helps transport iron from mother to child. It will be used to treat AIDS patients and as a supplement for infant formula.

Some scientists believe that transgenic research is similar to the discovery of domestication and selective breeding. Domestic animals were bred specifically to improve certain natural characteristics of a species. Cows were bred to give more milk, greyhounds were bred for speed, and sheep were bred for softer wool. Domestication and selective breeding rely on genes already in the animal, but transgenic breeding takes foreign genes from one species and puts them into another.

The first step is to locate the gene sequence on human DNA that contains the information to make the protein. Then the gene is cut off the human DNA strand and attached to a section of a cow's DNA, in the same manner as film is cut and spliced together. The altered DNA is placed inside a cow egg, and allowed to grow.

What matures is an animal like Herman, who now has the protein-making gene sequence in every cell in his body. This sequence will be naturally inherited by the offspring. Performing this procedure correctly on just a few animals can produce an entire protein-making herd.

Herman is not the only transgenic animal that has been bred. Goats and sheep are also being used, because scientists have discovered that a milking animal's mammary glands can be effective protein-making factories. They naturally produce and deliver proteins in milk that would go to the animal's own young, but the genetically altered protein would be extracted from the milk and given to human patients. Goats are good milkers and frequently give birth to twins and triplets that mature quickly, which rapidly increases the size of the herd and the amount of milk being produced.

Prior to the development of transgenic animals, human proteins were extracted from human sources or made in bacteria cultures. However, most proteins do not grow well in such cultures, and sometimes the yield from an entire vat would be so small as to be measured in a thousandth of a gram, which costs thousands of dollars.

Proteins extracted from sheeps' or goats' milk are measured in grams per liter, and the output is very good. A farm lab in Edinburgh, Scotland, raises transgenic sheep whose milk contains up to thirty-five grams per liter of a human blood protein called human alpha-1 antitrypsin. It will be used to replace the blood protein in patients who do not have enough and are at risk of developing life-threatening emphysema and other lung diseases.

Tissue plasminogen activator (t-PA) is another human protein important in treating a variety of human clotting disorders, such as hemophilia, AIDS, and chemotherapy-treated cancer. Transgenic goats now carry the gene to make human t-PA, as much as seven grams per liter of milk. A herd of 125 dairy goats may be able to produce the protein, instead of a $100 million factory built for that same purpose.

Transgenic animals have also revolutionized disease research.

Scientists can design laboratory mice with conditions that mimic or duplicate human diseases such as AIDS, diabetes, cancer, cystic fibrosis, and sickle-cell anemia. The mice become models in which researchers can study the disease and how it works, and researchers can test drugs on human tumor cells without actually putting people at risk.

Medicines may someday be grown on the farm, and so might replacement body parts. In the future, a doctor may be able to order a transgenic pig when an organ is needed. Pigs are being bred to contain genetically engineered "human" organs because they are easy to breed and their organs are about the same size as human organs.

The donor pigs are given human genes that tell the pig's body to make special human proteins that will protect the organs from being rejected when transplanted into a human body. The xenograft—an organ transplanted from one species into another—could fill the void of donor organs for patients awaiting a new heart, liver, or kidney. Donor pigs are way in the future, but already more than fifty bioengineered pigs have been bred in the barnyard/laboratories of Cambridge University, in England, and at Washington University School of Medicine, in St. Louis.

It is estimated that in the future ninety thousand pigs could provide enough organs for all Americans who need them. That is only one tenth of one percent of all the pigs that are currently being killed for food.[10]

Tobacco plants and rubber trees have also been experimented with to see if they can be altered to produce necessary drugs that once were expensively manufactured, or extracted from rare and endangered plants. New methods of bioengineering will also make it possible to grow vaccines, according to Dr. Michael Wilson at the Scottish Crop Research Institute.

"It may sound fanciful to say you can vaccinate yourself against a disease by plucking a banana off a tree and eating it, but this advance [in technology] makes it perfectly feasible."[11] In the future, transgenic technology might be an environmentally sound alternative to stripping the land in search of medicines.

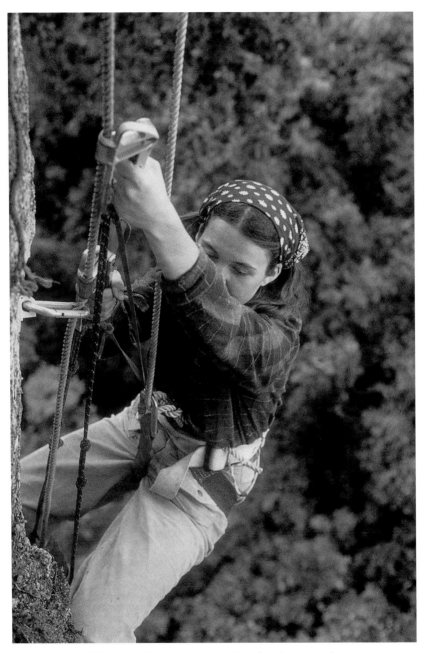

Often an ethnobotonist searching for plant samples
in the rain forest must climb trees to reach the canopy.

❧ *10* ❧

RAIN FOREST
REMEDIES

*I*n September 1987, John Burley, a British botanist, spent four weeks in the rain forest of Sarawak, Malaysia. He collected 136 different plant species for the NCI to test, which it did in 1991. A botanist never knows what unassuming-looking plant will be important, and Burley had no idea that one of his plants would prove successful during the HIV screening. It was a tree called *Calophyllum lanigerum*, a member of the gum-producing tree family, which Burley remembered collecting near a river in southern Sarawak. The tree was nothing special to look at. It stood fifty feet high and was less than two feet thick; nevertheless, it contained a compound that, in a test tube, appeared to protect human cells completely from the AIDS virus. The NCI chemists isolated eight different compounds from the tree, one of which was the anti-HIV substance they called calanolide A.[1]

A team from the University of Illinois, in Chicago, was sent back to Sarawak to collect more samples from this wonder tree. When they arrived in the area near the Batang Kayan River where Burley had collected his samples, all they found was a stump. The area, like most of Asia, was being cleared of trees to make way for farm- and pastureland. In the nearby forest, the botany team searched, but could not find another tree of the same species. Because of the immense biodiversity of the rain forest, trees rarely grow in solid stands as they do in forests in the United States. Trees of identical species might be miles apart. The team came back empty-handed.

It appeared that a miracle cure for AIDS had slipped through scientists' fingers. The tree stump sent a chilling reminder to chemical prospectors about the fate of the rain forests if steps are not taken to preserve them. The director of the Illinois team, Djaja Soejarto, was not satisfied with the situation. He went to see the pathetic stump for himself and to try to find another *Calophyllum* tree. Like his team members, Soejarto could not identify the same species, but he did find a variation that was remarkably similar. Quickly, it was tested. This new tree contained a compound almost identical to calanolide A, and the team called it costatolide.[2] Costatolide is not as powerful as the original compound, but it will have to do while plant hunters continue to look for the tree stump's next of kin.

Near a beach in the Philippines, a botanist from the Smithsonian Institution collected a sample of seaweed. Testing revealed that it had unusual potency for killing cancer cells. More was collected, but for some unknown reason, the sample did not exhibit the same activity. A large mass of the seaweed was again identified farther out at sea and was scheduled for collection by a research team. Before it could be collected, a typhoon hit and wiped out the entire mass. Marine biologists are still looking for the cancer-killing seaweed.

This pattern of finding promising chemical compounds only to have them disappear is happening more and more often. Here today, gone tomorrow is the botanist's dismal real-ity. No one can prevent a typhoon, but the loss of the rain forest is something that can be stopped. Rain forest land the size of Florida is being burned and cleared each year. The extinction rate is estimated at a chilling 27,000 species every year—74 species a day that will never again grace this earth.[3] Ethnobotanists ask themselves: at this rate, when another deadly disease attacks the human race, will there be sufficient natural resources to find the cure?

Malaria plagued the world until quinine was found. When quinine-resistant parasites appeared, a drug called chloroquinine replaced it, but now, in some parts of the world, chloroquinine has lost its effectiveness. Nature has once again provided an answer, a Chinese plant called artemisia. But what will happen when parasites develop resistance to artemisia? Will there be another drug to replace it, or will our biodiversity be so depleted that the next malarial drug no longer exists?

People living in the United States, and in other industrialized countries, have to realize that what happens to the rain forests does indeed affect our lives. Many of our drugs are based on rain forest plants, and chances are good that more of our future drugs, especially AIDS treatments, will come out of the tropics as well. How do we ensure a future source of medicine? It can be done by protecting biodiversity, and by preserving traditional healers' knowledge.

PROTECTING BIODIVERSITY

The rain forests hold the majority of species on earth, and history has proved to us that those species are chemically rich and therefore medicinally valuable. Ethnobotanists are worried that in the time it takes to bring a drug to market, which is ten to twenty years, most of the world's rain forests will be gone, so a small group of scientists are uniting in an effort to interest developing countries in assessing their plants with an eye toward preserving and using them responsibly.

In 1992, the Earth Summit was held in Rio de Janeiro, Brazil, and two important treaties were signed: one regulates global warming, and the other protects biological diversity. Sadly, the United States was the only industrialized country that refused to sign the biodiversity treaty, on the grounds that the details of some of the policies were not specific enough.

Many countries, however, have taken the first step toward preserving their biodiversity by taking inventory of all the species. In 1989, the small Central American country of Costa Rica formed the National Institute of Biodiversity (INBio). It started with a small staff, with some of the most impressive biologists in the world as advisers. Their goal is to save species by taking inventory and then finding a way to use them. In a sense, they are making nature pay its own way. It is not a popular point of view in some respects, because it is unclear who owns the natural resources and who will benefit. INBio has trained nonscientists from all walks of life—homemakers, bus drivers, park rangers, and cooks—in collection of specimens and conservation. INBio is effectively showing the world that conservation can pay off, by using its biodiversity and by training its citizens in marketable conservation skills.

One of the largest pharmaceutical companies in the United States, Merck & Company, set a precedent when it became partners with INBio in 1991. Merck paid $1 million to INBio in exchange for exploration rights and biological samples from the Costa Rican rain forest. INBio will also get a percentage of the royalties from any product that is based on a discovery in that country. Other pharmaceutical companies are joining forces with conservation/research groups. Pfizer Pharmaceuticals contracted with the New York Botanical Garden to screen plants collected in the United States.

Thomas Eisner, who helped broker the INBio and Merck deal, would also like to protect a site in upstate New York that would be the first United States preserve specifically used for biodiversity studies and chemical prospecting in a temperate environment.[4] A pharmaceutical company would finance the deal, while scientists would do the prospecting. Eisner believes that successful business and conservation collaborations could open up a new way of protecting the environment. Nature, business, science and people would all win.

The NCI is turning to one-on-one collaboration with foreign countries, such as Brazil, Mexico, South Africa, and Pakistan, to develop their abilities to collect and screen for medicinal specimens. The NCI will provide the cancer cell lines for screening and will invite scientists to the NCI labs to watch their operations. The countries will do the collecting and screening and, in the event that a drug is found, the NCI would collaborate on its development.

One problem that exists is that we cannot base judgment about the value of a species on current limited knowledge. Prior to Fleming's penicillin experiments, modern people never knew the medicinal value of mold; similarly, Taxol was not known to be a cancer-killing agent until proper tests for cancer were developed. An extract that is tested by the NCI today and shows no or low activity may turn out to be a powerful drug for a disease for which we have yet to devise a test. Scientists warn that the biodiversity survey should not be used to determine what species are expendable or valuable. Someday there may be a new disease to deal with, and that job will be made more difficult if our drug sources have been badly diminished because we did not think they were valuable.

Once a medicinal source has been found, how can it be used without destroying the forests as cattle ranching or other industries have done? One way is to preserve the land where the plants grow wild. A supporter in this movement is Rosita Arvigo, of the Belizean Healers' Association. She and many other experts feel that native peoples should have more control over their own environment. After all, they have managed the rain forests this long, and who else is more qualified? One of Arvigo's jobs has included rescuing medicinal and rare plants from land scheduled to be bulldozed. The plants are dug up and transplanted in a nursery called Ix Chel Tropical Research Foundation, named after the Mayan goddess of healing. It is a park full of orphan medicinal plants that young shaman apprentices can study.

A larger reserve, Terra Nova, covers more than six thousand acres, and is located near the Cayo District in Belize. The first ethnobiomedical reserve in the world, it was established in 1993.[5] It is run by the Traditional Healers' Association, which oversees the reserve where many types of Mayan medicinal plants are tended and used by the healers and their students.

Another organization, founded by a surgeon, José Cabanillas, is the Ethnomedical Preservation Project, which will set up a reserve of its own to protect medicinal plants and to combine Western medicine and traditional medicine effectively. Cabanillas's concern is the loss of medicine, not for Western medical research but for the local people who depend on these remedies every day.[6] The focus is to strengthen traditional knowledge, not to replace it with Western medicines.

For millennia, healers have gathered medicinal plants by means of a sustainable harvest, which means that they collect only what is needed at a rate that allows plants to continue to reproduce. Experts believe that this can be done on a larger scale as well. Trees that are medicinally useful, such as the croton tree in the Amazon, are being grown on farms. In agroforestry, a new system of experimental farming, produce and medicinal crops are planted alongside rain forest trees. The tree roots grow deep and bind the soil, acting as a nutrient pump for the crops. The mix of trees and crops gives villages a source of income as well as food to eat. Some scientists warn, however, that the more land is brought under cultivation, the greater is the threat to biodiversity.[7] Prospecting for new chemical compounds should be done, but synthesizing a drug in the laboratory would take the pressure off the environment. This was seen in the case of the Pacific yew tree, when harvesting the trees threatened the species' survival.

❧ SHARING THE WEALTH ❧

Governments must learn that the rain forests are worth more standing than they are if they are cut down, but part of the problem has been that industrialized nations have viewed the Third World's natural resources as free for the taking. These countries are cash poor but biodiversity rich, and they are just now starting to realize that their natural products should not be taken out of their own countries without compensation. By placing a focus on the value of medicinal plants, debt-ridden nations can stop depending on short-term monetary gains associated with logging, cattle grazing, and cash cropping, and instead become financially stable by conserving their resources.

In the past, poor countries have not fared well in their dealings with Western companies. It was common for scientists to take large quantities of plant material for study without giving anything in return. Research is increasingly based on traditional knowledge of the land, plants, and sustainable harvesting, and it should be compensated for. The rights to knowledge are called intellectual property rights; unfortunately, this is a difficult concept to implement, because who is to say to what extent a person, community, or country should be compensated for knowledge?

One of the first companies to start involving the host country in decisions and a share of the profits was Shaman Pharmaceuticals.[8] This company believes that since the local communities are the primary source of their information and material, they should be the ones to be compensated. Tribal leaders and shamans are included in decisions about what happens in their forests. Many times, the exchange for knowledge might include a financial agreement and a share in the profits, but this exchange also might include short-term and long-term benefits, such as medical care for villages that are isolated. One village asked Shaman Pharmaceuticals to have its airstrip lengthened so that medical supplies and patients could be flown in and out.

Larger pharmaceutical companies are entering into this type of agreement also, and the NCI requires its collecting agencies to use a contractual document called a Letter of Collection to arrange collection and compensation with a foreign government. If a drug were to be patented, the company would be required to work out compensation with the country where the compound originated.

It seems as if the combined pharmaceutical and conservation effort is all about making money, and to some extent it is. Right or wrong, people tend to save only those things that have value. If we cannot place a value on the rain forest, it will surely be burned away as so much charcoal. Biodiversity-rich nations have to acknowledge the fact that they hold a great legacy in their boundaries, a natural resource that affects the entire planet, and if they can profit from a conservationally sound use of the natural products, then we will all benefit.

✆ THE LOSS OF MEDICINAL KNOWLEDGE ✆

Saving the trees from the bulldozer may be an easier task than saving the thousands of years' worth of unwritten medicinal knowledge that native cultures possess. Traditional ways have been seriously threatened since the first explorers broke the culture barrier, followed by violent foreign governments and by missionaries intent on changing people's beliefs, as well as by the natural processes of change that occur when cultures come in contact with each other. What concerns scientists is that this process has put traditional knowledge at risk of disappearing. For example, younger people, attracted to Western culture, do not want to be apprentices to the aging shamans or to learn the old ways. Mark Plotkin believes that "each time one of these medicine men dies, it is as if a library has gone up in flames."[9] Somebody must be there to carry on the tradition.

Ethnobotany's whole premise is preserving and learning this medicinal wisdom, but some people believe a more concerted effort is needed to help strengthen threatened cultures. For example, Mark Plotkin set up a program called Shaman's Apprentice: he takes his research notes and has them translated back into the traditional language so that they can be used by apprentices and others in the village. In another instance, Shaman Pharmaceuticals responded when a young man who had been chosen as the shaman's apprentice was forced to leave his village and work in a tea plantation to earn money for his family. Shaman Pharmaceuticals set up a fund so that the man did not have to leave, and he could earn money while learning from the most revered healer in the village. In India, a program called Medicine Woman teaches women how to conduct an inventory, use a plant press, and perform basic laboratory techniques. This system was designed to give women job skills as well as to perpetuate traditional ways.

Preserving traditional medical knowledge is a complex issue. How can cultures continue to grow and change, and yet maintain important knowledge that may benefit the scientific and medical world? Who should be involved in the effort to preserve this knowledge? It is a problem that Third World and industrialized countries, as well as scientists, healers, and pharmaceutical companies, are struggling to solve.

✎ Healing Earth ✎

It is difficult to discuss saving natural medicinal sources without talking about the larger issue of saving the environment. The two are connected, and the protection of natural medicines should give us a special reason to protect the earth as a whole. The Endangered Species Coalition has a publicity poster that illustrates this connection with a poster child, a girl who was cured of leukemia by the endangered rosy periwinkle. Another poster shows a woman living a healthy life because of Taxol made from the threatened Pacific yew tree. Dedicated people are rallying to save the environment, not for pharmaceutical companies to make new medicines—that is only a side benefit. They are doing it to protect all species, including humans, but they are often faced with government budget cuts that threaten to lift conservation laws, and an industrial society that continues to distance us from our roots.

People are linked to the earth as tightly as any other creatures, and our health is dependent on the health and preservation of other life on the planet. We cannot cure ourselves if we destroy the source of those cures. An ancient philosophy states that for every disease nature inflicts, nature will also provide a cure. Only by respecting the environment can we continue to discover medicines from nature.

Some Medicines From Plants

Medicine	Medical Use	Plant Source
aspirin	reduces pain, inflammation, and clotting	white willow tree
atropine	dilates the pupils of the eyes	belladonna
digitalis	heart medication	foxglove
d-tubocurarine	anesthetic	chrondrodendron (curare)
etoposide	cancer drug	mayapple
ipecac	induces vomiting	ipecac shrub
morphine	potent painkiller	opium poppy
quinine	combats malaria	cinchona tree
reserpine	lowers blood pressure	Indian snakeroot
Taxol	cancer drug	Pacific yew and English yew
vinblastine	treatment for Hodgkin's disease	rosy periwinkle
vincristine	treatment for childhood leukemia	rosy periwinkle

Some Medicines From Animals

Medicine	Medical Use	Animal Source
hemetin	prevents blood clots	Amazon leech
istatin	treatment for fungal infections	bacteria on shrimp eggs
squalamine	antibiotic	bacteria from dogfish shark
virapin	reduces pain and improves blood flow	bee venom

GLOSSARY

agroforestry—A method of farming in which crops are planted among forest trees.

alkaloid—A chemical compound that contains at least one nitrogen atom; found in many plants that have medicinal value.

antibiotic—A substance that kills or stops the growth of bacteria.

assay—A test to determine the characteristics, biological activity, and strength of a chemical compound.

bacteria—One-celled microscopic organisms that are simpler than plant or animal cells and do not have an organized nucleus.

biodiversity—The vast variety of all species on earth, including microorganisms, plants, and animals.

cancer—A malignant growth of abnormal cells that can form harmful tumors.

chemical prospecting—Seeking out and testing soil, plants, and animals for unknown chemical compounds.

entomologist—A scientist who studies insects.

ethnobotany—The study of the relationship between people and plants: how they are used for food, medicine, clothing, housing, and tools.

herb—An aromatic plant with fleshy leaves and little or no woody parts; a plant used for medicinal purposes.

herbarium—A museum that houses collections of plant specimens.

materia medica—All the medicinal substances used by a particular culture.

molecule—A chemical unit made up of two or more atoms held together by a chemical bond.

pharmaceutical—A manufactured medicinal drug.

pharmacology—The study and development of new drugs and their safety and effectiveness.

poultice—A moist, often warm, medicated substance on a cloth applied to sores or wounds.

shaman—In the Amazon it refers to a spiritual leader who also knows the medicinal abilities of plants; in other cultures it means a spiritual leader only.

steroid—A chemical compound that is a solid alcohol occurring naturally in plants and animals.

sustainable harvest—Taking from the environment at a rate that allows nature to replenish itself, maintaining a constant supply.

synthesize—To make a substance that does not occur naturally; to make in a lab.

therapeutic—Having healing abilities.

tonic—A substance that restores vigor and strength.

transgenic—The transfer of genetic material from one species to another.

voucher specimen—A whole plant or animal, or a portion of it, collected for study.

zoopharmacognosy—The study of animals and how they use plants as medicines.

SOURCE NOTES

CHAPTER 1

1. Mary Roach, "Secrets of the Shamans," *Discover* (November 1993): 60.

2. Ibid.

3. Christopher Joyce, *Earthly Goods* (Boston: Little, Brown, 1994), 213.

4. Ibid., 8.

5. Ibid., 19.

6. Paul Alan Cox and Michael J. Balick, "The Ethnobotanical Approach to Drug Discovery," *Scientific American* (June 1994): 82.

7. Ibid., 83.

8. Cathy Sears, "Jungle Potions," *American Health* (October 1992): 70.

9. O. Akerele, V. Heywood, and H. Synge, *Conservation of Medicinal Plants* (New York: Cambridge University Press, 1991), 1–362.

10. Thomas Burton, "Drug Company Looks to 'Witch Doctors' to Conjure Products," *Wall Street Journal*, 7 July 1994, A-1.

11. Jacqueline Cossmon, "Ethnobotany Accelerating Drug Discovery," Shaman Pharmaceuticals, April 1995, 3.

12. World Health Organization, Regional Office for the Western Pacific, *Research Guidelines for Evaluating the Safety and Efficacy of Herbal Medicines* (Manila: WHO, 1993).

13. Roach, "Secrets," 63.

14. Howard Facklam and Margery Facklam, *Plants* (Springfield, N.J.: Enslow Publishers, 1990), 73.

CHAPTER 2

1. Christopher Joyce, *Earthly Goods* (Boston: Little, Brown, 1994), 8.

2. Inge N. Dobell, ed., *Magic and Medicine of Plants* (Pleasantville, N.Y.: Reader's Digest, 1986), 51.

3. Ibid., 52.

4. Ralph S. Solecki, "Shanidar IV: A Neanderthal Flower Burial in Northern Iraq," *Science* (November 1975): 880.

5. Charles Marwick, "Growing Use of Medicinal Botanicals Forces Assessment By Drug Regulators," *Journal of the American Medical Association* (22 February 1995): 607.

6. Mark Bricklin, "On the Spice Route," *Prevention* (July 1992): 31.

7. Robert A. Barnett, "Gingko, Ginger, Garlic, Ginseng," *Remedy* (September 1996): 34.

8. Jean Seligman, Geoffrey Cowley, and Susan Miller, "Sex, Lies and Garlic," *Newsweek* (November 6, 1995): 65.

9. "Garlic Shuts Down Human Cancer Cells in Mice," *Cancer Biotechnology Weekly* (24 April 1995): 4.

10. Barnett, "Gingko," 38.

11. Seligman et al., "Sex," 65.

12. Joel Gurin, ed., "Herbal Roulette," *Consumer Reports* (November 1995): 699.

13. Center for Medical Consumers Inc., "Herbal Ecstacy Herbal Weight Loss," *HealthFacts* 21 (June 1996): 5.

14. Ibid.

CHAPTER 3

1. Margaret B. Kreig, *Green Medicine: The Search for Plants That Heal* (Chicago: Rand McNally, 1964), 207–222.
2. Ibid., 169–206.
3. Geoffrey Marks and William K. Beatty, *The Medical Garden* (New York: Charles Scribner's Sons, 1971), 57.
4. Ibid., 64.
5. Christopher Joyce, *Earthly Goods* (Boston: Little, Brown, 1994), 40–45.
6. Kreig, *Green Medicine* 272–292.

CHAPTER 4

1. Francine Jacobs, *Breakthrough: The Story of Penicillin* (New York: Dodd, Mead, 1985).
2. Margery Facklam and Howard Facklam, *Healing Drugs* (New York: Facts On File, 1992), 53.
3. Ibid., 54.
4. Ibid., 57.
5. Robert S. Boyd, " 'Outbreak' of Disease Not Altogether Hollywood Fantasy," *Buffalo News*, April 1995, H6.
6. Richard Saltus, "Flesh-eating Bug Killed My Mother in 20 Minutes," *American Health* (September 1994), 74.
7. Ibid., 75.
8. Boyd, " 'Outbreak,' " H6.
9. Donna Alvarado, "Era of Antibiotics May End Because Resistant Bacteria Are Proliferating," *Buffalo News*, 19 February 1995, H8.

CHAPTER 5

1. National Cancer Institute, "Cancer Facts," National Institutes of Health, May 1994, 1.
2. "Emergency Teams Sampling Destroyed Palms As Source of New Drugs," *AIDS Weekly* (14 September 1992), 9.
3. National Cancer Institute, 5.

4. Ibid.

5. Ibid.

6. Christopher Joyce, *Earthly Goods* (Boston: Little, Brown, 1994), 257–258.

7. Gordon Cragg, interview by author, October 1996.

CHAPTER 6

1. Konrad Spindler, *The Man in the Ice* (London: Weidenfeld and Nicolson, 1994), 87.

2. Hal Hartzell Jr., *The Yew Tree: A Thousand Whispers* (Eugene, Oregon: Hulogosi, 1991), 6.

3. William Shakespeare, *Macbeth*, 4.1. 28–29.

4. Hartzell, *Yew Tree*, 4–5.

5. Tom Junod, "Tree of Hope," *Life* (May 1992): 71.

6. Ibid.

7. Ibid.

8. William P. McGuire et al., "Taxol: A Unique Antieoplastic Agent with Significant Activity in Advanced Ovarian Epithelial Neoplasms," *Annals of Internal Medicine* (1989): 273.

9. Ross C. Donehower and Eric K. Rowinsky, "Paclitaxel," *Cancer Principles and Practice of Oncology* (October 1994), 5.

10. Douglas Daly, "Tree of Life," *Audubon* (March–April 1992): 80.

11. Ibid., 81.

12. "Scientists Studying Alternative Source of Taxol," *Cancer Weekly* (September 1992): 3.

13. Hartzell, *Yew Tree*, 228–231.

14. Gail Dutton, "Uncommon Pathway to Uncommon Drugs," *The World and I* (August 1995), 154.

CHAPTER 7

1. Douglas Barasch, "Fishing for Drugs," *American Health* (March 1990): 20.

2. Michelle Kearns, "Davy Jones' Medicine Chest: Chemists Pursue a Treasure Trove of Drugs from the Deep," *Omni* (June 1994): 12.

3. Ibid.

4. "Anti-Cancer Drugs from Marine Invertebrate Symbiotic Bacteria," *Cancer Researcher Weekly* (June 1993): 9.

5. A. J. Hostetler, "Bioluminescence of Fish Offers a Potential Weapon Against Bacteria Resistant to Drugs," *Buffalo News*, 12 February 1994, H6.

6. National Cancer Institute, "Cancer Facts," National Institutes of Health, May 1994: 5.

7. William Sargent, *The Year of the Crab: Marine Animals in Modern Medicine* (New York: W. W. Norton, 1987), 71–81.

8. "Fishing for a Cancer Cure," *Discover* (September 1988): 10.

9. Catherine Dodd, "Shark Therapy," *Discover* (April 1996): 51.

CHAPTER 8

1. Blaine Harden, " 'Little Boogers' Make a Comeback," *Buffalo News*, April 1995.

2. Elizabeth DeVita, "Bloodcurdling Therapies," *American Health* (October 1994), 13.

3. Roy T. Sawyer, "In Search of the Giant Amazon Leech," *Natural History* (December 1990), 66–67.

4. May R. Berenbaum, *Bugs in the System* (Reading, Mass: Helix Books, 1995), 173.

5. Ibid.

6. Randi Hutter Epstein, "Maggots Are Employed As 'Nature's Remedy,'" *Buffalo News* (July 1995), F6.

7. Ibid.

8. Thomas Eisner, interview by author, July 1995.

9. Ibid.

10. Berenbaum, *Bugs*, 171–172.

11. James F. Scheer, "Propolis: The Bees' Gift to Human Health," *Better Nutrition for Today's Living* (March 1994), 38.

12. Katie Rodgers, "Back to Our Roots: Searching for New Drugs in the Rain Forest," *Drug Topics* (January 1995): 57.

13. Mark W. Moffett, "Poison-Dart Frogs, Lurid and Lethal," *National Geographic Magazine* 187 (May 1995): 98.

CHAPTER *9*

1. Ron Cowen, "Medicine on the Wild Side: Animals May Rely on a Natural Pharmacy," *Science News* 138 (November 3, 1990): 280.

2. Ann Gibbons, "Plants of the Apes," *Science News* (February 1992): 21.

3. James Grisanzio, "The Monkey's Medicine Chest," *Technology Review* (August–September 1995): 14.

4. Cowen, "Medicine," 280.

5. Grisanzio, "Monkey," 14.

6. D'Arcy Jenish, "Threatened Animals: Poachers Are Supplying an Oriental Demand," *Maclean's* 102 (7 August 1989): 44.

7. Ibid.

8. Ibid., 45.

9. Anne Simon Moffat, "Transgenic Animals May Be Down on the Pharm," *Science* (October 1991): 35.

10. "Pigs for Transplants," *American Health* (June 1994): 9.

11. "Crop Scientists Make Vaccines Grow on Trees," *Cancer Biotechnology Weekly* (January 1996): 17.

CHAPTER *10*

1. "Researchers Still Searching for Lost AIDS Tree," *AIDS Weekly* (May 1993): 13.

2. Christopher Joyce, *Earthly Goods* (Boston: Little, Brown, 1994), 252.

3. Ibid., 97.

4. Jon R. Luoma, "Better Living Through Botany," *Audubon* (March–April 1996): 24.

5. Rosita Arvigo and Nadine Epstein, *Sastun* (New York: Harper-Collins, 1994), 180.

6. Katie Rodgers, "Back to Our Roots: Searching for New Drugs in the Rain Forest," *Drug Topics* (January 1995): 58.

7. Madhusree Mukerjee, "Sowing Where You Reap," *Scientific American* (May 1996): 24.

8. Steven R. King, Thomas Carlson, and Katy Moran, "Biological Diversity, Indigenous Knowledge, Drug Discovery and Intellectual Property Rights," in *Indigenous Knowledge and Intellectual Property Rights*, ed. S. Brush and D. Stabinsky (1993), 173.

9. Mark J. Plotkin, *Tales of a Shaman's Apprentice* (New York: Penguin Books, 1993).

FURTHER READING

Arvigo, Rosita, and Nadine Epstein. *Sastun*. New York: Harper-Collins, 1994.

Berenbaum, May R. *Bugs in the System*. Boston: Helix Books, 1995.

Dobell, Inge N., ed. *Magic and Medicine of Plants*. Pleasantville, N.Y.: Reader's Digest, 1986.

Facklam, Margery, and Howard Facklam. *Healing Drugs: The History of Pharmacology*. New York: Facts On File, 1992.

Hartzell, Hal Jr. *The Yew Tree: A Thousand Whispers*. Eugene, Ore.: Hulogosi, 1991.

Joyce, Christopher. *Earthly Goods: Medicine Hunting in the Rainforest*. Boston: Little, Brown, 1994.

Kreig, Margaret. *Green Medicine*. Chicago: Rand McNally, 1964.

Plotkin, Mark J. *Tales of a Shaman's Apprentice*. New York: Penguin Books, 1993.

Sargent, William. *The Year of the Crab: Marine Animals in Modern Medicine*. New York: W. W. Norton, 1987.

Serrentino, Jo. *How Natural Remedies Work*. Washington, D.C.: Hartley and Marks, 1991.

Wilson, E. O. *The Diversity of Life*. Cambridge, Mass.: Harvard University Press, 1992.

INDEX